AMERICAN JOURNAL of PUBLIC HEALTH
FEBRUARY 2023
Issue 2

AJPH

A PUBLICATION OF THE
AMERICAN PUBLIC HEALTH ASSOCIATION

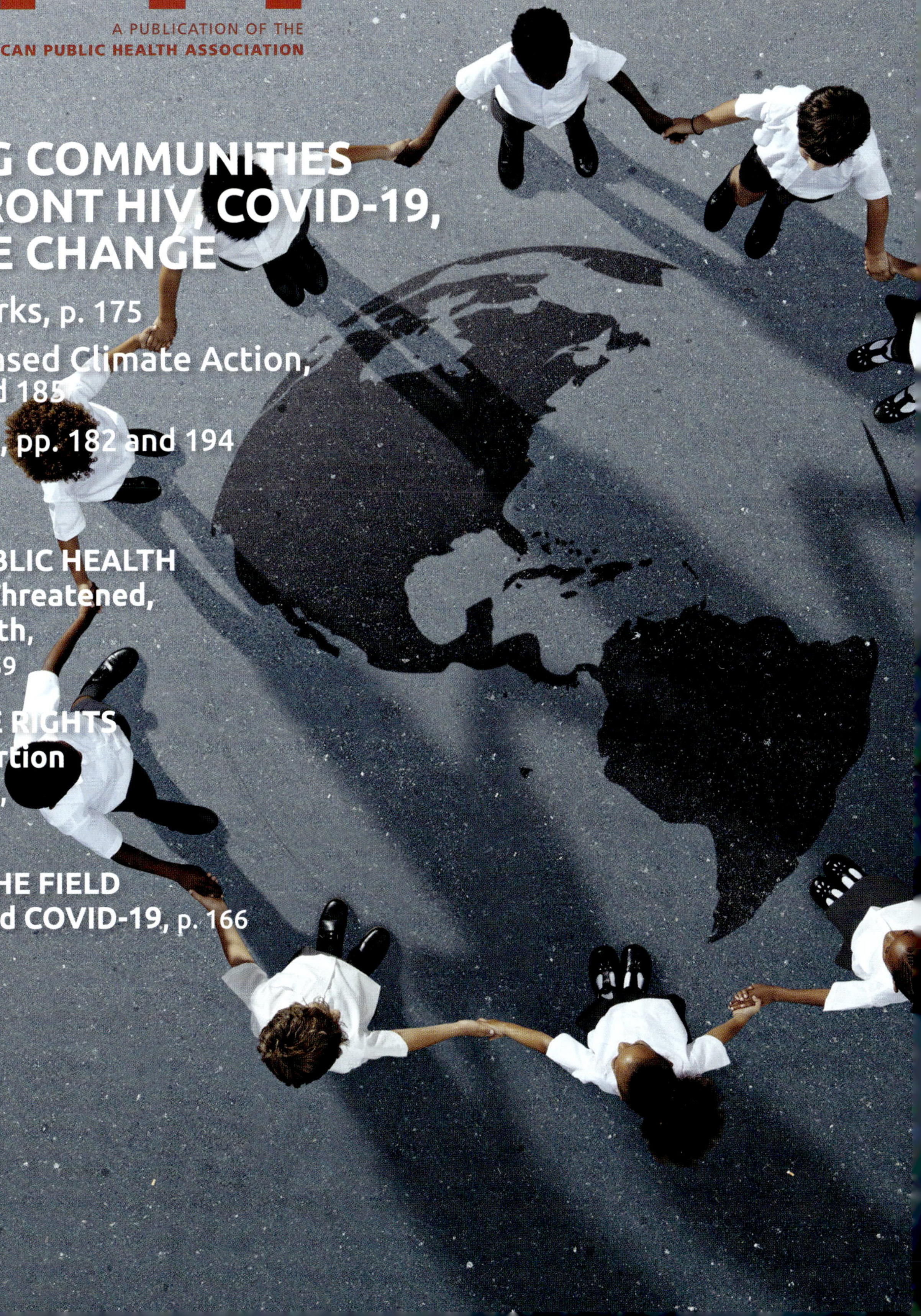

ENGAGING COMMUNITIES TO CONFRONT HIV, COVID-19, & CLIMATE CHANGE

New Frameworks, p. 175

Community-Based Climate Action, pp. 177, 179, and 185

Health Justice, pp. 182 and 194

Also in this issue:

PEACE AND PUBLIC HEALTH
When Peace Is Threatened, So Is Pubic Health, pp. 132 and 146–159

REPRODUCTIVE RIGHTS
Medication Abortion "Reversal" Laws, pp. 138 and 202

NOTES FROM THE FIELD
Farmworkers and COVID-19, p. 166

APHA
AMERICAN PUBLIC HEALTH ASSOCIATION
For science. For action. For health.

AJPH®, published monthly, is the official Journal of the American Public Health Association®, 800 I St NW, Washington, DC 20001-3710; (202) 777- APHA; TDD (202) 777-2500. APHA is a nongovernmental professional society founded in 1872, representing all disciplines and specialties in public health.

The *American Journal of Public Health*® (*AJPH*) (print ISSN: 0090-0036; electronic ISSN: 1541- 0048), first published in 1911, is the official journal of the American Public Health Association® (APHA). The oldest and largest organization of public health professionals in the world, APHA represents approximately 30 000 members from more than 50 occupations of public health.

Submissions: Visit www.editorialmanager.com/ajph or ajph.edmgr.com for online manuscript preparation and submission guidelines. Contributions of original unpublished research, social science analyses, scholarly essays, critical commentaries, departments, and letters to the editor are welcome. Questions? Write ajph.submissions@apha.org or call APHA at (202) 777-2469.

Print plus online subscriptions: Institutional price (print copy with online access for a single institution and all authorized users, regardless of geographic location) varies by size of organization and ranges from $993–$1445 for US organizations, and $1073–$1526 for international organizations (air delivery); multiple campuses not permitted without special arrangement. Details of the tiered pricing system at https://subscriptionoffice.com/pages/apha-landing-page. To order, write apha.subscriptions@apha.org.

Online only subscriptions: Institutional price for one institution and its authorized users (regardless of geographic location) is $878–$1307. To order, write apha.subscriptions@apha.org. For academic consortia or multisite corporate subscriptions, contact apha.subscriptions@apha.org.

Print-only subscriptions: Institutional price is US $701, $782 international.

Back print issues: A limited number of print issues are for sale. Single copies are US $49, $55 international (air delivery). Shipping included; prepay only. To order, write apha.subscriptions@apha.org.

Reprints: For prices and ordering information on 50 or more reprints, check the Reprints section at www.ajph.org. To order smaller quantities of reprints (rush delivery), use the "Purchase Article" link on the article site itself.

Electronic access: Online articles more than 10 years old are available free for personal use at www.ajph.org. Recent articles are available through pay-per-view: single PDF article for $24, single issue access for 24 hours for $33, or entire site access for 24 hours for $38.

Postal information: Periodicals postage paid at Washington, DC, and additional mailing offices. Postmaster: Send address changes to American Journal of Public Health, 800 I St NW, Washington, DC 20001-3710.

Address changes: Send to AJPH, Membership Department (members) or AJPH Subscriptions (subscribers), APHA, 800 I St NW, Washington, DC 20001-3710. Or write to membership.mail@apha. org (members) or apha.subscriptions@apha.org (subscribers).

Advertising: For pricing and other information, see www.ajph.org. Please write to ashell.alston@apha.org or call (202) 777-2470 for other advertising opportunities. Ask about special exhibit packages and sponsorships. Acceptance of advertising by the *Journal* does not imply endorsement of products.

Indexes: Publications that index or abstract articles from AJPH include the following: Ageline, Assia (Applied Social Science Index and Abstracts), Biological Abstracts, Chemical Abstracts, CINAHL, Criminal Justice Abstracts, EMBASE, EMCare, Environmental Abstracts, e-psyche, ERIC, ETOH (Alcohol and Alcohol Problems Science Database), Excerpta Medica, Food Science and Technology, General Science Index, Grateful Med, Hospital Literature Index, Human Resources Abstracts, International Pharmaceutical Abstracts (IPA), Medline, Physical Education Index, Pollution Abstracts, Psychological Abstracts, PsychINFO, Safety Science Abstracts, Sage Family Studies Abstracts, Sage Human Resources Abstracts, Science Citation Index, SCOPUS, SIIC Data Bases, Social Work Research and Abstracts, and Statistical Reference Index (SRI)/LexisNexis.

Medscape Publishers' Circle

AJPH

A PUBLICATION OF THE
AMERICAN PUBLIC HEALTH ASSOCIATION

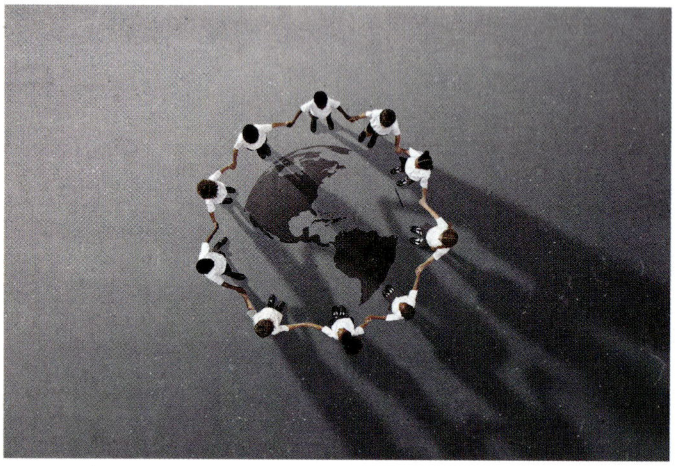

COVER: Peace is fundamental for health and public health advocacy. Sustainable and effective public health responses are directly related to a baseline level of both direct and structural violence. In this issue of the journal, we explore threats to peace across three dimensions: direct violence, pockets of fragility, and forced displacement and migration.

Cover concept and selection by Aleisha Kropf. Photo by Klaus Vedfelt, courtesy of Getty Images. Printed with permission.

Support for this issue was provided by a grant from the Robert Wood Johnson Foundation.

APHA
AMERICAN PUBLIC HEALTH ASSOCIATION
For science. For action. For health.

Promoting public health research, policy, practice, and education is the *AJPH* mission. As we widen our scope to embrace global issues, we also sharpen our focus to support the needs of public health practitioners. We invite contributions of original unpublished research, opinion and commentary, and letters to the editor.

The *Journal* is printed on acid-free recycled paper.

OPEN ACCESS ONLINE ONLY PODCAST DATA SUPPLEMENT AVAILABLE

EDITOR'S CHOICE

132 When Peace Is Threatened, So Is Public Health
L. Vahedi, C. Harb, S. Tate, A. Nguyen, T. Ellis, S. Woolsey, and J. J. Suen

BOOKS & MEDIA

133 Public Health and War: Hope Among the Horrors?
O. Razum and L. Wandschneider

OPINIONS, IDEAS, & PRACTICE

EDITORIALS

136 A Global South Perspective: The Intersection of COVID-19 and Intimate Partner Violence
R. J. Ferreira and F. Buttell

138 Countering the Antiscience of Abortion Regulation
P. Skuster

141 Revisiting Patient Engagement and Empowerment Within the NIMHD Health Disparity Framework
M. R. T. Spencer and J. Chen

144 Women, Life, Freedom: A Public Health of Consequence, February 2023
F. Kapadia

STUDENT THINK TANK

146 Peace Beyond the Binary: A Creative Intersectional Perspective on Global Forced Displacement
A. Gillespie

149 The Peace Exchange: Physical and Psychological Sacrifices of Military Personnel From Historically Marginalized Backgrounds
A. McCullers

152 Honoring Dignity in Violent Times
B. Zimmerman

155 Forgotten People in Forgotten Places: The Uncounted Costs of Conflict
A. J. Blum

158 Pathways to Peace and Public Health Equity Among Women and Children in Conflict Zones: The Case of Northern Uganda
S. Awor

IMAGES OF HEALTH

160 The Visibility of Evictions (an Image of Health)
E. Persaud

NOTES FROM THE FIELD

162 Treating Hepatitis C in Individuals With Previous Incarceration: The Veterans Health Administration, 2012–2019
L. Hawks, E. A. Wang, A. A. Butt, S. Crystal, D. K. McInnes, V. L. Re III, E. J. Cartwright, L. B. Puglisi, L. Y. K. Haque, J. K. Lim, A. C. Justice, and K. A. McGinnis

166 CDC-Supported National Network of Farmworker-Serving Organizations to Mitigate COVID-19
B. Boggess, S. Prager, J. M. Lincoln, N. E. Foss, E. Kissam, S. Partida, and A. R. Lainz

170 A COVID-19 Vaccination Program to Promote Uptake and Equity for People Experiencing Homelessness in Los Angeles County
A. D. Rosen, A. Senturia, I. Howerton, E. U. Kantrim, V. Evans, T. Malluche, J. Miller, M. Gonzalez, B. Robie, C. L. Shover, A. H. Chang, H. Behforouz, A. Nguyen, and E. H. Thomas

ENVIRONMENTAL AND HEALTH JUSTICE

175 New Frameworks for Engaging Communities to Confront HIV, COVID-19, and Climate Change Health Inequities
J. I. Levy and L. Bowleg

177 Understanding Challenges to Health Equity in Climate Action and Land Use Planning
M. Méndez and M. E. Zuñiga

179 Redefining the Quest for Health Equity in the Era of Climate Crisis
A. R. Riley

182 Health Justice in the Context of Health and Human Rights
L. Ferguson

RESEARCH & ANALYSIS

ENVIRONMENTAL AND HEALTH JUSTICE

185 Advancing Health Equity in Community-Based Climate Action: From Concept to Practice
B. L. Cole, I. D. Rosario, A. Hendricks, and D. P. Eisenman

194 Health Justice: A Framework for Mitigating the Impacts of HIV and COVID-19 on Disproportionately Affected Communities
S. Alang and O. Blackstock

LAW & ETHICS

202 Medication Abortion "Reversal" Laws: How Unsound Science Paved the Way for Dangerous Abortion Policy
S. K. Redd, R. AbiSamra, S. C. Blake, K. A. Komro, R. Neal, W. S. Rice, and K. S. Hall

POLICY

213 Insurance-Based Discrimination Reports and Access to Care Among Nonelderly US Adults, 2011–2019
K. T. Call, G. Alarcon-Espinoza, N. S. M. Arthur, and R. Jones-Webb

OPEN-THEMED RESEARCH

224 Rural–Urban Disparities in Adverse Maternal Outcomes in the United States, 2016–2019
K. A. Harrington, N. A. Cameron, K. Culler, W. A. Grobman, and S. S. Khan

228 The COVID-19 Pandemic, Socioeconomic Effects, and Intimate Partner Violence Against Women: A Population-Based Cohort Study in 2020, Iran
R. Fereidooni, J. Mootz, R. Sabaei, K. Khoshnood, S. T. Heydari, M. J. Moradian, E. Taherifard, M. Nasirian, and H. Molavi Vardanjani

BACKMATTER

OTHER DEPARTMENTS

238 Subscription Form

When Peace Is Threatened, So Is Public Health

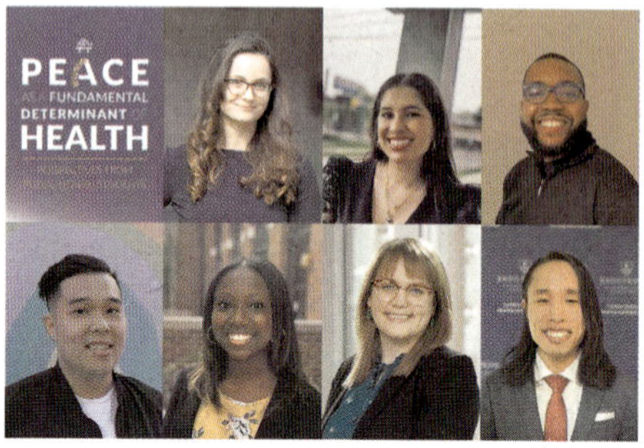

The commitment to preventing disease, promoting health, and prolonging life at the population level has shifted efforts away from individualizing health disparities to understanding how social and structural determinants shape individual health outcomes. However, there is less-explicit focus on what conditions shape socio-political structures. A baseline level of peace, defined as the absence of both direct and structural violence (https://tinyurl.com/2s3jhh5h), is often an unstated assumption that underscores our ability to mount effective and sustainable public health responses.

The tenure of the 2022 *AJPH* Student Think Tank occurred during several paradigm-shifting socio-political events (the COVID-19 pandemic, highly visible and racialized violence in the United States, the civil war in Ethiopia, the femicide of Mahsa Jina Amini in Iran, and the war in Ukraine just to name a few), which challenged us to critically reflect on whether the socio-political environments where public health is practiced have truly ever been peaceful.

The nexus between health and peace is not new; in 1981, the World Health Assembly's Resolution stated, "the preservation and promotion of peace is the most significant factor for the attainment of health for all" (https://bit.ly/3HD3yVw). While there is an urgent need to conceptualize peace as a fundamental determinant of health, certain forms of direct and structural violence have become part of the zeitgeist.

When violence becomes normalized, it hampers the ability to recognize that the absence of peace anywhere poses global threats to public health everywhere. For example, the legacy of armed conflict in the Democratic Republic of the Congo has eroded medical and public health infrastructure, rendering Congolese populations vulnerable to emerging infectious diseases that can now spread internationally faster than ever before (https://tinyurl.com/52t7ja6w). Furthermore, despite the United States maintaining the world's highest gross domestic product (https://tinyurl.com/mr2d7fkj), US maternal mortality rates rank among the highest globally, with Black women experiencing three times the risk of death compared with their White counterparts (https://tinyurl.com/2bwryeca), thereby yielding intergenerational adversities. The direct violence from armed conflict and the structural disparities that cause the premature mortality of Black women illustrate that when peace is threatened, so is public health.

We conceptualize threats to peace across three dimensions. First, the presence of direct violence in the form of war and conflict between and within nations has a profound effect on whether environments sustain life or exacerbate premature morbidity and mortality. Second, high-income countries can have "pockets of fragility," wherein subpopulations experience a disproportionate disease burden. Third, forced displacement and migration, either within a country or across international borders, can yield intergenerational health adversities at the intersection of gender, class, and race.

To highlight our conceptualization of the peace–health nexus, we present diverse student perspectives and experiences on the theme of peace as a fundamental determinant of health (see pp. 146–159). The selected submissions engage critically with the most pressing public health issues at the crossroads of peace and health. The submissions collectively emphasize that the absence of peace anywhere and among any group threatens us all. Without peace, public health cannot reach its goals of preventing disease, promoting health, and prolonging life. It is time for the public health community to declare explicitly that peace is fundamental for health and to advocate accordingly. AJPH

Luissa Vahedi, MSc
Clara Harb, MPH, MA
Shokhari Tate, MPH
Antony Nguyen, BA
Tyana Ellis, PhD, MSPH
Summer Woolsey, MPH, TTS
Jonathan J. Suen, AuD
2022 AJPH Student Think Tank

DOI: https://doi.org/10.2105/AJPH.2022.307185

12 Years Ago

The New Left and Public Health

We continue wrestling with the politics of "community"—a term invoked frequently (and often mystically) yet imprecisely in public health—and the associated search for sources of transformation in health provision. Historical and present efforts related to government health insurance have been propelled mainly by middle-class reformers, not more popular constituencies. With some exceptions, mass organizing around health equality remains difficult.

From AJPH, February 2011, pp. 247–248

45 Years Ago

Consumer-Based Boards of Health Centers

Consumers need to be involved in the larger health care system, not just in the governance of local facilities such as health centers. This would provide new power bases and open up communication channels between higher levels in the health care system and consumers on local levels. The effect would be that local consumer board members would have access to information other than that channeled through the traditional professional channels. . . . It may be that consumer board members should have some identifiable constituency. This could take the form of official representation of other relevant community organizations, thereby providing a power base as well as relevant organizational experience for potential board members. If this occurs, providers and other professionals should be prepared for an increase in conflict, as consumers would now come to the board with vested interests and increased self-confidence.

From AJPH, June 1978, p. 581

Public Health and War: Hope Among the Horrors?

Oliver Razum, MD, MSc, and Lisa Wandschneider, MSc

ABOUT THE AUTHORS

Oliver Razum and Lisa Wandschneider are with the Department of Epidemiology and International Public Health, School of Public Health, and the Research Institute Social Cohesion (RISC), Bielefeld University, Bielefeld, Germany.

See also Cole et al., p. 185, Ferguson, p. 182, Levy and Bowleg, p. 175, Mendéz and Zuñiga p. 177, and Riley, p. 179.

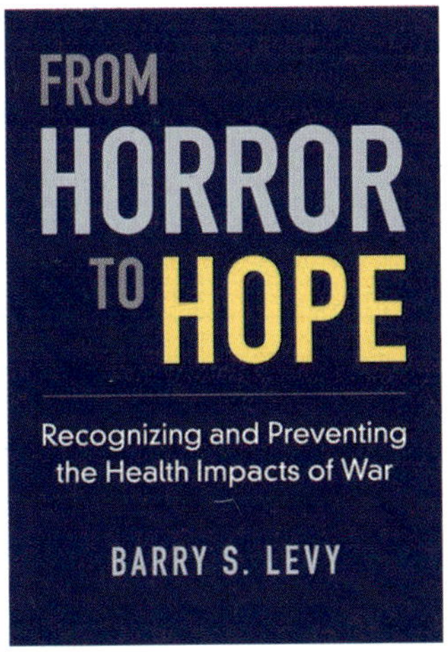

From Horror to Hope: Recognizing and Preventing the Health Impacts of War
By Barry S. Levy
New York, NY, and Oxford, UK; Oxford University Press; 2022.
304 pp; $55.
ISBN: 978-0-19755-864-5 (paperback).

"War is a man-made public health problem," argued the Turkish Medical Association when the Turkish army attacked Kurdish areas in Afrin, Syria.[1] The American Public Health Association (APHA) placed war "among the most important public health problems of the last 100 years," with "little evidence that its importance is waning."[2] Barry S. Levy, in his new book *From Horror to Hope: Recognizing and Preventing the Health Impacts of War*, agrees, and speaks of war as a "public health catastrophe." What more can be said?

TIMELY AND ACCOMPLISHED

A lot more, as Levy's work shows. Levy is a physician with the Department of Public Health and Community Medicine, Tufts University School of Medicine, and former APHA president. His publications cover social injustice, environmental health, climate change, terrorism, and war, from a public health perspective. *From Horror to Hope* brings together what has preoccupied Levy throughout his professional life. He describes how war affects population health in different forms and dimensions, ranging from injuries, mental and reproductive health, to (non)-communicable diseases, and he identifies subpopulations at particular risk, from children to military personnel. He covers the effects of different types of weapons, as well as legal and ethical aspects of war. Importantly, Levy proposes what role public health professionals can play in preventing war and promoting peace. His book will be of interest to public health students and practitioners wishing to obtain an overview of these long-neglected topics.

The breadth of the topics Levy covers is impressive. In some places, more in-depth technical details could inform the actions and practices of public health professionals. For example, there is an extensive list of chemical agents used in weapons of mass destruction, yet it remains open how their health effects can be treated, and what public health resources this would require. The section on nuclear weapons rightly focuses on the risk of total mutual destruction. Yet Russia's President Putin, his invasion of Ukraine failing, may resort to "low-yield" tactical nuclear warheads. Levy does not provide much detail of a public health response—which would be quite different in the two scenarios. It would range from explicitly warning the public that no health workers and infrastructure will be left to assist survivors of an all-out nuclear war to detailed advice on how to avoid physical and radiation injury, building on the dubious "duck and cover" campaigns in the 1950s. Public health workers face a dilemma here: claiming that they can alleviate a population's suffering after a nuclear attack would be unethical—but so would declining to prepare for nuclear war.

MORE DILEMMAS AND AMBIGUITIES

Dilemmas and ambiguities abound in the context of 21st century wars—for example, those relating to when a war starts, and what constitutes a weapon. Levy describes new weapons such as drones and cyberattacks. One could add here weaponized health communication, which may be deployed well before military action is taken. Broniatowski et al. provide evidence of Russian Twitter bots and Internet trolls amplifying a debate on measles vaccination in Ukraine in 2014, thereby compounding vaccine supply problems.[3] Vaccine uptake among Ukrainian children declined dramatically, as Figure 1 shows, followed by an outbreak with tens of thousands of cases in 2018 and 2019. Substantial public health resources were and are required to make up for the ensuing loss of trust, extending to the COVID-19 pandemic.

An additional public health dilemma, which is often neglected, pertains to "othering" processes in times of war. To legitimize weapon use, territorial war, or regime change, the attacking party will construct an "other," such as a purported Nazi regime in Ukraine as Russia's justification for its war of aggression; or a regime allegedly hoarding weapons of mass destruction, as in the second Iraq war. A core element of othering processes is a power asymmetry.[4] This asymmetry manifests in terms of military, economic, or knowledge power. In a war of aggression, the aggressor makes use of these power asymmetries, and subsequently attacks in the respective fields—not necessarily, or not only, in the military field.

In othering processes, the equal worth of individuals is challenged from a position of power. In a war, othering leads to dehumanization, which rarely remains one-sided, even in an asymmetric war.[5] In Ukraine, for example, the enemy forces are called "russians" (with a small "r") and labeled as nonhuman, monstrous creatures. Additional forms of othering associated with war scenarios include the detainment of population groups in camps.[4] In these scenarios, public health practitioners face yet another dilemma. On the one

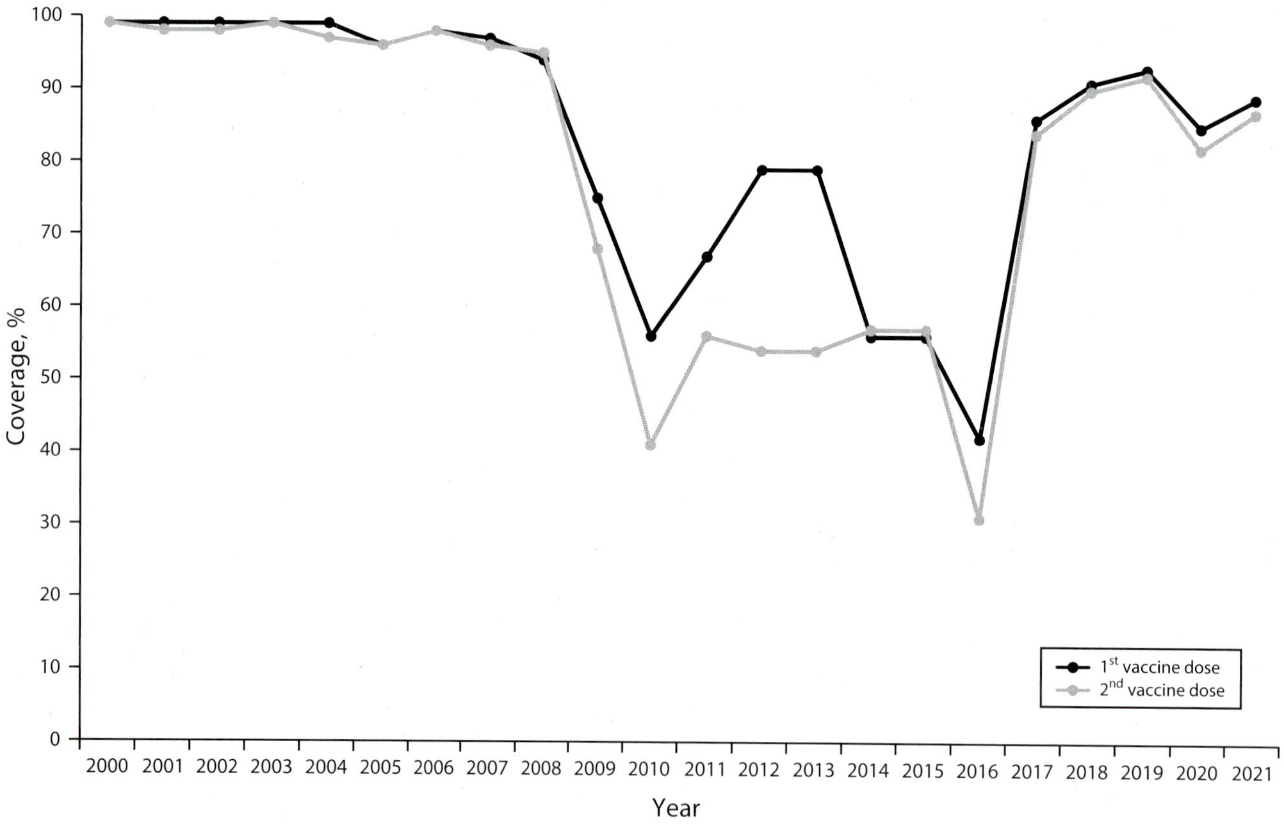

FIGURE 1— Measles Vaccination Coverage Among Children in Ukraine in Percentages, 2000–2021

Note. Black line: first vaccine dose; gray line: second vaccine dose.
Source. WHO Immunization Dashboard Ukraine (https://immunizationdata.who.int/pages/profiles/ukr.html).

hand, they need to identify, publicize, and help to reduce economic and knowledge asymmetries between groups and between nations, emphasizing again and again the equal value of all human beings, and to reject attempts at othering particular groups. On the other hand, they have to concede that nations need defense systems that are able to balance asymmetries in military power to protect populations and their health from aggressors, such as Russia, that ruthlessly break international law. Democratic societies with a realist view of world politics will conceive a well-funded military as a means of primary prevention of war. Even when striving for disarmament, they will concede, for the time being, a need for the very weapons, including nuclear weapons, that inevitably turn war into a public health catastrophe.

CHALLENGES

Levy prefers other means of preventing war, which he discusses in the concluding chapter. Diplomacy and reconciliation are core elements of promoting peace, and Levy recommends, for example, "speaking truth to power." Yet activists against war incur high personal risks. Members of the Turkish Medical Association were sentenced to prison terms after their protests and freed only after international expressions of solidarity.[1,6] Russian citizens who protest against their government's war in Ukraine lack a comparable visibility, institutional backup, and supportive lobby.

That does not mean that public health scientists and practitioners should give up idealist positions, or that they should stop actively opposing war. First, they need to continue documenting direct and indirect war-related health consequences, as Levy and colleagues such as Victor W. Seidel have impressively done over the past decades.[7] Levy portrays several more doctors, activists, and scientists in his book who contribute to this endeavor. Second, public health scientists and practitioners must find a balance between pointing out the limitations they are facing, being unable to protect population health in all-out wars; and explaining means of mitigation and prevention. And third, they need to identify, and aim at reducing, othering processes in and between societies early on, thus helping to stop divisiveness and hatred.

"From Horror to Hope" is a fitting motto these days, when the future looks precarious: humanity may well eradicate itself—and many other species—through unmitigated climate change or in an all-out war. Far too little has been done to protect the future.[8] Public health scientists and practitioners ought to spend substantially more time and resources assessing and communicating these horrors and their health consequences—helping to keep them at bay, and thereby investing in the future from a position of hope. In other words, they should follow Barry Levy's remarkable example. AJPH

CORRESPONDENCE

Correspondence should be sent to Oliver Razum, Department of Epidemiology and International Public Health, School of Public Health, Bielefeld University, PO Box 10 01 31, D-33501 Bielefeld, Germany (e-mail: oliver.razum@uni-bielefeld.de). Reprints can be ordered at http://www.ajph.org by clicking the "Reprints" link.

PUBLICATION INFORMATION

Full Citation: Razum O, Wandschneider L. Public health and war: hope among the horrors? *Am J Public Health*. 2023;113(2):133–135.

Acceptance Date: October 31, 2022.

DOI: https://doi.org/10.2105/AJPH.2022.307168

CONTRIBUTORS

O. Razum drafted the manuscript. L. Wandschneider contributed individual sections and revised the entire manuscript for critical intellectual content. Both authors read and approved the final manuscript.

ACKNOWLEDGMENTS

O. Razum's work is partly funded by the German Research Foundation (DFG), project FOR2928 PH-LENS, subproject OTHER.

CONFLICTS OF INTEREST

Both authors declare that they have no conflicts of interest.

REFERENCES

1. Razum O, Barros H, Buckingham R, et al. Is war a man-made public health problem? *Lancet*. 2019; 394(10209):1613. https://doi.org/10.1016/S0140-6736(19)31900-2
2. American Public Health Association. The role of public health practitioners, academics, and advocates in relation to armed conflict and war. APHA Policy Statement 20095. 2009. Available at: https://www.apha.org/policies-and-advocacy/public-health-policy-statements/policy-database/2014/07/22/13/29/the-role-of-public-health-practitioners-academics-and-advocates-in-relation-to-armed-conflict. Accessed November 21, 2022.
3. Broniatowski DA, Jamison AM, Qi S, et al. Weaponized health communication: Twitter bots and Russian trolls amplify the vaccine debate. *Am J Public Health*. 2018;108(10):1378–1384. https://doi.org/10.2105/AJPH.2018.304567
4. Razum O, Dawson A, Eckenwiler L, Wild V, eds. *Refugee Camps in Europe and Australia: An Interdisciplinary Critique*. New York, NY: Palgrave Macmillan; 2022. https://doi.org/10.1007/978-3-031-12877-6
5. Bruneau E, Kteily N. The enemy as animal: symmetric dehumanization during asymmetric warfare. *PLoS One*. 2017;12(7):e0181422. https://doi.org/10.1371/journal.pone.0181422
6. Rubenstein L. *Perilous Medicine: The Struggle to Protect Health Care From the Violence of War*. New York, NY: Columbia University Press; 2021.
7. Levy BS, Sidel VW. Documenting the effects of armed conflict on population health. *Annu Rev Public Health*. 2016;37(1):205–218. https://doi.org/10.1146/annurev-publhealth-032315-021913
8. MacAskill W. The beginning of history: surviving the era of catastrophic risk. *Foreign Aff*. 2022; 101(5):10–24.

A Global South Perspective: The Intersection of COVID-19 and Intimate Partner Violence

Regardt J. Ferreira, PhD, and Fred Buttell, LCSW, PhD

ABOUT THE AUTHORS

Regardt J. Ferreira is with the Disaster Resilience Leadership Academy, Tulane School of Social Work, New Orleans, LA, and Stellenbosch University, Stellenbosch, South Africa. Fred Buttell is with the Tulane School of Social Work and the University of the Free State, Bloemfontein, South Africa.

See also Alang and Blackstock, p. 194, Fereidooni et al., p. 228, and Kapadia, p. 144.

AJPH February 2023, Vol 113, No. 2

Intimate partner violence (IPV), formerly termed domestic violence (DV), is a pernicious social problem that has proven to be difficult to target and treat effectively. Most of what we know about IPV, including ideas about its causes, consequences, treatments, and interventions (including outcomes), comes from a Western paradigm.

WESTERN MODALITIES

Beginning with the battered women's shelter movement in the 1970s in England, domestic violence policies really got traction in the late 1980s in the United States with the majority of the states passing legislation that criminalized it. These laws either encouraged (proarrest) or required (mandatory) police responding to DV calls to identify the abuser and arrest him (most were gender-specific at the time of their passing). These laws were crafted to move past the Castle Doctrine, which essentially viewed the state's right to intrude on a citizen's life as stopping at the front door, because a man's home was his castle.[1]

Predictably, this seismic shift in policy led to a large increase in the number of men arrested, prosecuted, and convicted of DV offenses in the criminal justice system. This groundswell of men being processed into the criminal justice system threatened to cripple an already overtaxed system, and it was quickly acknowledged that paying a small fine (misdemeanor DV) or going to jail (typically 30 days for misdemeanor DV) would do little to equip these men with a skill set to prevent future types of similar behavior. As a consequence, court-referred treatment and intervention programs quickly emerged as an alternative to fines or jail time. This, in turn, led to a large body of research being devoted to evaluating the outcomes of these batterer intervention programs.

The red thread that connects all of these disparate parts of IPV for the past three decades is the feminist paradigm. Emerging from the beginning of the shelter movement, the primary explanation for the cause of IPV was that we exist in a patriarchal culture in which violence against women (i.e., heterosexual male violence directed toward a female intimate partner) is both sanctioned and part of the socialization process. This view is foundational to understanding the etiology of why men assault women and led to the development of a dominant intervention program for batterers that was codified in state laws around the United States (i.e., the Duluth program) and was also codified at the federal level with the passing of the Violence Against Women Act of 1994 (most recently reauthorized in 2022).

HEARING THE VOICE FROM THE GLOBAL SOUTH

Despite the wide-ranging and easily accessible information available on IPV in Western countries, there is a significant delta between that body of work and information available from countries in the Global South. To begin the process of rectifying this imbalance, in 2021, the World Health Organization (WHO) released its report on global IPV rates for 2018 and reported that the lifetime rate for women who will experience physical violence, sexual violence, or both is 26% for women aged 15 years and older.[2] The report is comprehensive and breaks this rate down by regions of the world. Viewing the occurrence of IPV through a feminist lens, it can be anticipated that more-patriarchal countries, where women have fewer rights and freedoms, will have higher-than-average rates of IPV.

For the purposes of this WHO report, Iran is categorized in the Eastern

Mediterranean Region, and the lifetime rate of IPV for that region is 31%. The rates of IPV reported by the WHO serve as important background information for the IPV rates revealed in this study. Making matters more complicated, the COVID-19 pandemic has proven to be challenging on many fronts, with IPV taking center stage as a major global public health concern, in response to pandemic-related strategies like lockdowns.[3,4]

In this issue of *AJPH*, Fereidooni et al. (http://bit.ly/3NV9xG8) undertook an investigation that examined the prevalence of IPV during COVID-19 among Iranian women. We want to laud the authors for undertaking such an important study, given the scant literature on IPV within the context of pandemics generally and out of the Global South and Iran specifically. The study reveals that the IPV rate for its sample of Iranian women was 54.2% in 2019 (prepandemic) and 65.4% during the pandemic.

The rates identified in the study are two times higher than those reported for the region, but it should be noted that these figures include sexual violence, physical violence, and psychological violence, while the WHO data exclude psychological violence. However, the findings are consistent with one of the few other studies of IPV among Iranian women. In a study involving a sample of 240 women developed using multistage random sampling, Mohammadbeigi et al.[5] reported an IPV rate of 28.8% for physical and sexual violence and an overall rate of IPV including psychological violence of 80%.

Taken as a whole, the findings from the Fereidooni et al. study are consistent with what one might expect for a country like Iran that is widely viewed as oppressive for women, but they are important for several reasons. First, they provide empirical evidence for what would seem intuitively true from a feminist perspective. Second, they provide empirical data documenting the impact COVID-19 public health prevention measures had on increasing IPV risk for women, with an emphasis on the Global South. Third, they found that a male partner becoming unemployed increased IPV risk for his female partner and that socioeconomic status served as a protective factor for women, both of which are true in Western countries.[6] The Fereidooni et al. study serves to further the argument made in other studies that we should unify efforts to address violence against women by providing yet more evidence that IPV is a global public health problem that is not bound by hemisphere, continent, or region.[7] *AJPH*

CORRESPONDENCE

Correspondence may be sent to Regardt Ferreira, School of Social Work, Tulane University, 127 Elk Place, New Orleans, LA 70112-2627 (e-mail: rferrei@tulane.edu). Reprints can be ordered at https://ajph.org by clicking the "Reprints" link.

PUBLICATION INFORMATION

Full Citation: Ferreira RJ, Buttell F. A Global South perspective: the intersection of COVID-19 and intimate partner violence. *Am J Public Health*. 2023;113(2):136–137.

Acceptance Date: October 2, 2022.

DOI: https://doi.org/10.2105/AJPH.2022.307144

CONTRIBUTORS

Authors discussed and contributed to the article where needed.

ACKNOWLEDGMENTS

Funding for publication was provided, in part, by Tulane's Supporting Impactful Publications (SIP) Program.

CONFLICTS OF INTEREST

The authors report that they have no conflicts of interest.

REFERENCES

1. Jansen S, Nugent-Borakove ME. Expansions to the Castle Doctrine: implications for policy and practice. Washington, DC: National District Attorneys Association, American Prosecutors Research Institute; 2016.
2. Violence against women prevalence estimates, 2018: global, regional and national prevalence estimates for intimate partner violence against women and global and regional prevalence estimates for non-partner sexual violence against women. Geneva, Switzerland: World Health Organization; 2021.
3. Gosangi B, Park H, Thomas R, et al. Exacerbation of physical intimate partner violence during COVID-19 pandemic. *Radiology*. 2021;298(1): E38–E45. https://doi.org/10.1148/radiol.2020202866
4. Buttell F, Ferreira RJ. The hidden disaster of COVID-19: intimate partner violence. *Psychol Trauma*. 2020;12(suppl 1):S197–S198. https://doi.org/10.1037/tra0000646
5. Mohammadbeigi A, Sajadi M, Ahmadli R, et al. Intimate partner violence against Iranian women. *Natl Med J India*. 2019;32(2):67–71. https://doi.org/10.4103/0970-258X.275343
6. Alonso-Borrego C, Carrasco R. Employment and the risk of domestic violence: does the breadwinner's gender matter? *Applied Economics* 2017;49: 5074–5091. https://doi.org/10.1080/00036846.2017.1299103
7. Ferreira RJ. Climate change, resilience, and trauma: course of action through research, policy, and practice. *Traumatology*. 2020;26(3):246–247. https://doi.org/10.1037/trm0000282

Countering the Antiscience of Abortion Regulation

Patty Skuster, JD, MPP

ABOUT THE AUTHOR

The author is with the James E. Beasley School of Law, Temple University, Philadelphia, PA.

See also Redd et al., p. 202.

On an array of health concerns, policymakers have rejected science in favor of lawmaking based on ideology, politics, and religion to the detriment of public health. This is particularly true of stigmatized health areas such as reproductive health and, especially, abortion care.

Before the Supreme Court decision in *Dobbs v. Jackson Women's Health Organization*, state lawmakers who were determined to legally restrict abortion enacted laws with the purpose of impeding abortion care. As legislators bound by constitutional protections for the right to abortion, they could not ban abortion outright. Antiabortion lawmakers instead enacted laws that reject scientific evidence to discourage and create obstacles for both abortion providers and patients seeking abortions. Among the many types of antiscientific abortion regulations are medication abortion "reversal" laws. In this issue of *AJPH*, Redd et al. (p. 202) longitudinally examine these types of laws.

Medication abortion "reversal" is an untested and experimental treatment to stop the abortion process for patients who have undergone a medication abortion. Redd et al. note that, since 2015, 14 states have enacted laws requiring that patients be told about medication abortion reversal in the counseling process during an abortion, despite the lack of scientific basis for the treatment. Medication abortion reversal laws have primarily been enacted in states with legislatures that are hostile to abortion rights. Indeed, the authors note that legislatures in 11 of the 14 states with such laws have also enacted abortion bans.

With the rise of outright bans in abortion-hostile states after the *Dobbs* decision, medication abortion reversal laws on their own are likely to have less impact. However, attention to these and other antiscientific abortion laws remains critical to research and to ensuring access to abortion care. The Redd et al. findings highlight the urgent need to track and counter antiscience state abortion laws subsequent to the end of federal constitutional abortion rights.

TOWARD EVIDENCE-BASED ABORTION REGULATION

While abortion bans came into force in the weeks and months after the *Dobbs* decision, so did a surge in political will to protect abortion among abortion-supportive policymakers. As they demonstrate their commitment to abortion rights, public authorities should work to counter and repeal medication abortion reversal laws and the many other antiscience abortion laws in effect.

The abortion law situation in the United States has become extraordinarily complex since the *Dobbs* decision. Approximately half of US states have legislated bans on abortions that either are currently in force or have been temporarily blocked pending litigation. Policymakers have reformed laws to improve access. Interjurisdictional legal conflicts will usher in new areas of unprecedented legal complexity.[1] In many states where abortion is legal, obstacles to abortion remain because of laws enacted by antiabortion legislatures or because abortion-supportive legislators have voted for laws not based on evidence.

Abortion-supportive lawmakers indicate a greater willingness to forward laws and policies to protect abortion access in response to state abortion bans. Prosecutors have vowed not to enforce restrictive abortion laws. Municipal authorities have allocated public funding for abortion[2] and taken steps to protect abortion care.[3] States and municipalities have enacted shield laws to block cooperation with law enforcement agencies from other jurisdictions for the purpose of prosecuting abortion.[4] The federal government took steps to ensure that abortion would be provided in emergency cases according to federal law in states where abortion bans are in place.[5]

In addition, lawmakers who wish to support abortion access should work to repeal antiscience abortion laws, particularly in abortion-supportive legislatures. In the nearly 50 years during which the right to abortion was constitutionally protected in the United States, state lawmakers proliferated requirements for abortion care that

AJPH February 2023, Vol 113, No. 2

were not based on scientific evidence. These requirements numbered more than 1000 throughout the United States and included mandatory waiting periods, prohibitions on public funding for abortion, qualification requirements for abortion providers, and facility requirements, often accompanied by criminal penalties for noncompliance.[6]

For guidance on reform toward abortion regulation based on scientific evidence, lawmakers can look to the World Health Organization guideline on safe abortion.[7] The safe abortion guideline offers recommendations for abortion regulation based on systematic reviews of scientific evidence. Among other recommendations, the guideline calls for abortion to be available on the request of the pregnant person, calls for public financing of abortion, and recommends against mandatory waiting periods. The guideline recommends self-managed medication abortion up to 12 weeks of gestation and calls for removal of all criminal penalties for abortion.

TRACKING ABORTION LAWS

To understand the full scope of the need for reform and rigorously study antiscientific abortion laws across the United States after *Dobbs*, researchers must systematically collect and track legal data on abortion. Redd et al. demonstrate both the utility and the complexity of tracking state abortion laws. For a variety of audiences—abortion researchers, institutions working to expand access, and lawyers and advocates working toward reform—an accurate representation of abortion law over time will prove indispensable in this new era of chaotic application of laws.

Redd et al. developed a coding scheme to examine specific characteristics of medication abortion reversal laws and recorded information about time and geography for each of the laws. Coding allowed them to categorize laws according to their characteristics. This approach is a type of policy surveillance: systematic, scientific collection and analysis of laws of public health significance. Policy surveillance consists of methods for creating legal and policy data suitable for use in rigorous evaluation studies as well as for individuals and groups working to increase access to abortion care and reform abortion laws and policies.[8,9]

The sheer number and complexity of antiscience abortion laws call for scalable methods for analysis that can be applied to a larger number and scope of abortion laws and policies. The Center for Public Health Law Research has developed methods for systematic policy surveillance that can be scaled to accommodate a large body of state-level abortion law. For example, researchers have used policy surveillance methods and resources available through the center to rigorously assess laws regulating abortion facilities, including measures for quality control.[10] More recently, researchers have compiled a data set that provides a high-level overview of state abortion restrictions and protections enacted after the *Dobbs* decision.[11] For targeted law reform efforts, rigorous scientific study, and more informed abortion programming, such methods should be deployed to the full range of state and federal abortion laws.

CONCLUSION

The legal landscape for abortion in the United States shifted dramatically and suddenly on June 24, 2022, when the Supreme Court issued its opinion in *Dobbs v. Jackson Women's Health Organization*. Although state-level bans represent a major piece of the abortion regulation puzzle, a tangle of antiscientific state abortion laws remain. As Redd et al. demonstrate, informed policymaking and thorough research demand rigorous surveillance of antiscience abortion regulations. AJPH

CORRESPONDENCE

Correspondence should be sent to Patty Skuster, JD, MPP, Temple University Beasley School of Law, 1719 N Broad St, Philadelphia, PA 19122 (e-mail: patty.skuster@temple.edu). Reprints can be ordered at http://www.ajph.org by clicking the "Reprints" link.

PUBLICATION INFORMATION

Full Citation: Skuster P. Countering the antiscience of abortion regulation. *Am J Public Health*. 2023;113(2):138–140.

Acceptance Date: November 15, 2022.

DOI: https://doi.org/10.2105/AJPH.2022.307176

CONFLICTS OF INTEREST

The author has no conflicts of interest to declare.

REFERENCES

1. Cohen D, Donley G, Rebouche R. The new abortion battleground. Available at: https://scholarship.law.pitt.edu/cgi/viewcontent.cgi?article=1515&context=fac_articles. Accessed November 11, 2022.
2. New York City Council. Speaker Adrienne Adams, first-ever women majority New York City Council announce largest commitment of municipal funds by any city in US to support increased access to abortion care. Available at: https://council.nyc.gov/press/2022/09/13/2254. Accessed November 11, 2022.
3. Philadelphia City Council. Councilmembers Gym, Brooks, Gauthier announce legislative package to defend abortion access in Philadelphia. Available at: https://phlcouncil.com/councilmembers-gym-brooks-gauthier-announce-legislative-package-to-defend-abortion-access-in-philadelphia. Accessed November 11, 2022.
4. Florey K. Dobbs and the civil dimension of extraterritorial abortion regulation. *New York Univ Law Rev*. 2022; Epub ahead of print. https://doi.org/10.2139/ssrn.4172494
5. Centers for Medicare & Medicaid Services. Reinforcement of EMTALA obligations specific to patients who are pregnant or are experiencing pregnancy loss. Available at: https://www.cms.gov/medicareprovider-enrollment-and-certification surveycertificationgeninfopolicy-and-memos-states-and/reinforcement-emtala-obligations-specific-

patients-who-are-pregnant-or-are-experiencing-pregnancy-0. Accessed October 21, 2022.

6. Nash E. State policy trends 2021: the worst year for abortion rights in almost half a century. Available at: https://www.guttmacher.org/article/2021/12/state-policy-trends-2021-worst-year-abortion-rights-almost-half-century. Accessed October 21, 2022.
7. *Abortion Care Guideline*. Geneva, Switzerland: World Health Organization; 2022.
8. Burris S, Hitchcock L, Ibrahim J, et al. Policy surveillance: a vital public health practice comes of age. *J Health Polit Policy Law*. 2016;41(6):1151–1173. https://doi.org/10.1215/03616878-3665931
9. Skuster P, Menzel J, Ghorashi AR, et al. Policy surveillance for a global analysis of national abortion laws. *Sex Reprod Health Matters*. 2022;30(1):2064208. https://doi.org/10.1080/26410397.2022.2064208
10. Jones BS, Daniel S, Cloud LK. State law approaches to facility regulation of abortion and other office interventions. *Am J Public Health*. 2018;108(4):486–492. https://doi.org/10.2105/AJPH.2017.304278
11. Policy Surveillance Program. Post-Dobbs state abortion restrictions and protections. Available at: https://lawatlas.org/datasets/post-dobbs-state-abortion-restrictions-and-protections. Accessed November 11, 2022.

Revisiting Patient Engagement and Empowerment Within the NIMHD Health Disparity Framework

Merianne Rose T. Spencer, MPH, and Jie Chen, PhD

ABOUT THE AUTHORS

Merianne Rose T. Spencer and Jie Chen are with the Department of Health Policy and Management and the Hospital And Public Health InterdisciPlinarY Research (HAPPY) Laboratory, School of Public Health, University of Maryland, College Park.

See also Call et al., p. 213.

The US health care delivery system is at a pivotal juncture in addressing and reducing health disparities.[1] The COVID-19 pandemic has underscored how vulnerable patient populations in our US health care system are disproportionately experiencing barriers to accessing health care and receiving needed care.[2] Such health disparities, or rather "the health differences closely linked to economic, social, or environmental disadvantage [that] adversely affect groups of people who have systematically experienced greater social or economic obstacles in health," have revealed worse health outcomes by gender, race, ethnicity, socioeconomic status, religion, and other factors.[3(p6)] In this issue of *AJPH*, Call et al. (https://bit.ly/3B4RWXj) examined insurance-based discrimination in Minnesota. The study showed that patients who were uninsured or had public insurance experienced higher rates of insurance-based discrimination than patients with private insurance.

Framing this work within the National Institute on Minority Health and Disparities Research (NIMHD) Framework can offer insights into the study's observed findings.[1] According to the NIMHD Framework, health disparities persist across multiple domains (biological, behavioral, physical or built environment, sociocultural environment, and the health care system) that influence health outcomes at numerous levels (individual, interpersonal, community, and societal).[1] To adequately tackle multiple complexities and barriers to health—including insurance-based discrimination—policies must address both interpersonal and systemic issues in our country through policy reform, patient engagement, and overall better patient care for vulnerable and minority communities.

ENHANCING PATIENT–PHYSICIAN INTERACTIONS

The NIMHD Framework highlights various levels for improvement, starting at the individual and interpersonal levels. At the individual level, health literacy limitations and patients' responses to discrimination are stressors that have biological, behavioral, and interpersonal implications. Secondly, interpersonal levels of influence within the sociocultural environment and health care system, such as patient–provider (interpersonal) relationships and trust, as well as medical decision-making between patients and providers, are factors that cannot be overlooked. By focusing solely on one domain or level, we may fail to consider policies that can best lead to better-quality health care.

Thus, we must consider interventions starting with the patient–physician relationship. This relationship is bidirectional; therefore, approaches can be calibrated toward each group. Physicians have cited difficulties communicating with patients as one of the challenges faced in providing high-quality care.[4] Providing culturally sensitive personalized interventions can help sustain patient involvement in taking an active role in health care decision-making. As mentioned by Call et al., cultural competency training among physicians can improve the overall patient experience.

Additionally, the importance of patient activation, confidence, and empowerment—core components of the personalized patient activation and empowerment model for improved population health and reduction of racial and ethnic disparities—cannot be understated.[5] Patient empowerment, defined as the process through which people gain confidence and power over decisions and actions affecting their own health, calls for patient knowledge, participation, self-efficacy, and health literacy, and for facilitation of a workplace promoting empowerment.[6,7] By being encouraged to gain knowledge of their health conditions, treatment plans, or health care access from providers, patients can be more motivated to communicate about their health needs, express their health concerns,

AJPH February 2023, Vol 113, No. 2

and be activated and more engaged in their health care and with the providers with whom they interact.

Other approaches, such as improving patient–physician concordance and tackling language barriers and related issues inhibiting patient-driven health care, may enhance patient experiences. Studies have shown that physician–patient concordance improves health outcomes.[8] By using approaches that consider key elements between patients and physicians, we as a nation are taking important steps toward better health outcomes and quality health care.

PROMOTING POPULATION HEALTH

Although the interaction between patients and physicians is an important determinant of patient care, there are other factors that impede patient care, particularly for vulnerable populations. According to the NIMHD Framework, interventions must address numerous facets to enhance patient and provider experiences collaboratively.

The study by Call et al. captures one of the disparities observed at the societal level of the NIMHD Framework: insurance-based discrimination. The authors call attention to different reimbursement rates of public and private insurance. Indeed, Medicaid has a lower reimbursement rate than either Medicare or private health plans. The reimbursement rate of Medicaid is associated with physicians' decisions to accept new Medicaid patients, influencing access to high-quality patient care and health outcomes in the long run. Recent research suggested that closing the gap in reimbursement between Medicaid and private insurance would reduce disparities in access among adults by more than two thirds.[9] Access to high-quality health care and resources is a key component of social determinants of health, according to the NIMHD model.

To advance population health, pragmatic integration of the financing (e.g., reimbursement model), delivery (e.g., a coordinated health care system instead of siloed health care sectors), and health production (e.g., patient–physician relationship) sectors are needed in the United States. It is also important to acknowledge the interrelationship and interdependence of these components.

SYSTEMATIC APPROACH TO IMPROVE PATIENT-CENTERED CARE

Increasingly, policymakers, researchers, and health advocates have promulgated the quadruple aim as end goals for advancing health care delivery, where enhancing the patient experience, improving population health, reducing cost, and improving the work life of health care providers are fundamental paths to resolving health disparities and improving health care for all.[10] To achieve these aims, policies must center around patients. Recognizing the disparities in our system is one step toward achieving these aims; by actively enabling patients to participate in their care, we can move closer to equitable health care for all.

Incorporating patient–provider relationships into innovative health care delivery models, such as the patient-centered medical home (PCMH) model, presents an untapped opportunity to promote patient-centeredness and the patient experience. As suggested by its name, the PCMH model's core element centers around patient experience.[11] Implementing Consumer Assessment of Healthcare Providers and Systems surveys may help shed insight into modifiable factors of patient experiences, such as physician communication and the patient–provider relationship.

In addition, investments in care coordination practices and integration, along with innovative health care delivery models such as accountable care organizations, present an important opportunity for promoting continuity of care and patient experience.[12] As such, policies incentivizing approaches that enhance the patient–provider relationship can help tackle discrimination and promote health equity in the US health care system.

Future policies must look to the new normal post-COVID-19 era and consider innovative solutions that can enhance the patient experience while addressing structural-level barriers, social determinants of health, and other factors limiting access to affordable, quality health care. Understanding and enhancing the patient experience stems from addressing individual-level factors and factors affecting the environment, community, and organizations entrenched in delivering health care. AJPH

CORRESPONDENCE

Correspondence should be sent to Jie Chen, University of Maryland, Department of Health Policy and Management, 3310E School of Public Health Building, 4200 Valley Dr, College Park, MD 20742 (e-mail: jichen@umd.edu). Reprints can be ordered at http://www.ajph.org by clicking the "Reprints" link.

PUBLICATION INFORMATION

Full Citation: Spencer MRT, Chen J. Revisiting patient engagement and empowerment within the NIMHD health disparity framework. *Am J Public Health*. 2023;113(2):141–143.

Acceptance Date: November 3, 2022.

DOI: https://doi.org/10.2105/AJPH.2022.307170

CONTRIBUTORS

M. R. T. Spencer and J. Chen drafted and revised the manuscript.

ACKNOWLEDGMENTS

This study is supported by the National Institute on Aging (R01AG62315) and the National Institute on Minority Health and Health Disparities (R01MD011523).

CONFLICTS OF INTEREST

The authors have no known conflicts of interest.

REFERENCES

1. Alvidrez J, Castille D, Laude-Sharp M, Rosario A, Tabor D. The National Institute on Minority Health and Health Disparities Research Framework. *Am J Public Health.* 2019;109(suppl 1):S16–S20. https://doi.org/10.2105/AJPH.2018.304883
2. Clay SL, Woodson MJ, Mazurek K, Antonio B. Racial disparities and COVID-19: exploring the relationship between race/ethnicity, personal factors, health access/affordability, and conditions associated with an increased severity of COVID-19. *Race Soc Probl.* 2021;13(4):279–291. https://doi.org/10.1007/s12552-021-09320-9
3. Braveman P. What are health disparities and health equity? We need to be clear. *Public Health Rep.* 2014;129(suppl 2):5–8. https://doi.org/10.1177/00333549141291S203
4. Bustamante AV, Chen J. Lower barriers to primary care after the implementation of the Affordable Care Act in the United States of America. *Rev Panam Salud Publica.* 2018;42:e106. https://doi.org/10.26633/RPSP.2018.106
5. Chen J, Mullins CD, Novak P, Thomas SB. Personalized strategies to activate and empower patients in health care and reduce health disparities. *Health Educ Behav.* 2016;43(1):25–34. https://doi.org/10.1177/1090198115579415
6. Aujoulat I, Marcolongo R, Bonadiman L, Deccache A. Reconsidering patient empowerment in chronic illness: a critique of models of self-efficacy and bodily control. *Soc Sci Med.* 2008;66(5):1228–1239. https://doi.org/10.1016/j.socscimed.2007.11.034
7. Greene J, Hibbard JH, Sacks R, Overton V, Parrotta CD. When patient activation levels change, health outcomes and costs change, too. *Health Aff (Millwood).* 2015;34(3):431–437. https://doi.org/10.1377/hlthaff.2014.0452
8. Shen MJ, Peterson EB, Costas-Muñiz R, et al. The effects of race and racial concordance on patient–physician communication: a systematic review of the literature. *J Racial Ethn Health Disparities.* 2018;5(1):117–140. https://doi.org/10.1007/s40615-017-0350-4
9. Alexander D, Schnell M. The impacts of physician payments on patient access, use, and health. National Bureau of Economic Research Working Paper Series 26095. July 2019. Available at: https://www.nber.org/papers/w26095. Accessed October 31, 2022.
10. Bodenheimer T, Sinsky C. From triple to quadruple aim: care of the patient requires care of the provider. *Ann Fam Med.* 2014;12(6):573–576. https://doi.org/10.1370/afm.1713
11. Martsolf GR, Alexander JA, Shi Y, et al. The patient-centered medical home and patient experience. *Health Serv Res.* 2012;47(6):2273–2295. https://doi.org/10.1111/j.1475-6773.2012.01429.x
12. Barath D, Amaize A, Chen J. Accountable care organizations and preventable hospitalizations among patients with depression. *Am J Prev Med.* 2020;59(1):e1–e10. https://doi.org/10.1016/j.amepre.2020.01.028

Women, Life, Freedom: A Public Health of Consequence, February 2023

Farzana Kapadia, PhD, MPH

ABOUT THE AUTHOR

Farzana Kapadia is deputy editor of AJPH *and a professor of epidemiology at the School of Global Public Health, New York University, New York, NY.*

See also Alang and Blackstock, p. 194, Fereidooni et al., p. 228, and Ferreira and Buttell, p. 136.

AJPH February 2023, Vol 113, No. 2

The 2021 UN Women report "Measuring the Shadow Pandemic: Violence Against Women During COVID-19," with data from more than 16 000 women across 13 countries, confirms that since the start of the COVID-19 pandemic, both incidence and prevalence of violence against women (VAW) have increased, worsening an already existing crisis (https://bit.ly/3EDbfZF). Pandemic restrictions and lockdowns forced women into extended periods of isolation with their abusers as well as created a series of economic and social disruptions that likely played a role in exacerbating experiences of VAW during this time. The loss of employment and loss or reduction of wages for both women and their partners, the shuttering of schools, and the restrictions on movement outside the home, coupled with lack of privacy to contact police, support groups, family, and friends for assistance played critical roles in increasing exposure to all forms of VAW—physical, sexual, verbal, and psychological.

INTIMATE PARTNER VIOLENCE AGAINST WOMEN

In the UN Women report, a pooled average of 45% of women, ranging from 80% in Kenya to 25% in Paraguay, reported direct experience or knowledge of someone who experienced violence since the onset of the pandemic. More than two thirds of women, ranging from 92% in Kenya to 33% in Kyrgyzstan, reported that physical and verbal abuse by a spouse or partner had become more common in their community during the pandemic. Importantly, the economic and financial fallout resulting from the pandemic have exacerbated food insecurity (up to 58%) and reduced the likelihood of feeling safe in public settings (20%) for women across these 13 countries. Across the board, women who became unemployed during the pandemic were more likely to report experiencing violence, feeling less safe at home, and feeling less safe walking out alone in public spaces at night compared with employed women. These estimates of direct and indirect experiences with and knowledge of VAW are strong indicators of the degree to which gender-based social, cultural, economic, and political inequalities are so very deeply entrenched within and across our societies and cultures. And it is the pervasiveness and persistence of these inequalities coupled with discriminatory norms that allow VAW to continue and be considered an acceptable form of social control over women.

It is against this backdrop of increasing VAW that we must consider the work by Fereidooni et al. (p. 228), who examined changes in intimate partner violence (IPV) among 2300 women living in Isfahan, Iran. While acknowledging the significant methodological challenges in undertaking such a study, the findings of this study are alarming given the current political, economic, and social situation with respect to the rights of women in Iran. Specifically, the prevalence of IPV, including physical, psychological, and sexual violence, increased from 54.2% before the pandemic to 65.4% after the pandemic. Reinforcing the findings of the UN Women report, all women in this sample who reported losing their jobs reported experiencing IPV, and the odds of experiencing IPV were staggeringly high among those who had lost their job or had a partner who had lost their job compared with those who did not.

The addition of economic shocks in an environment where women's rights are already severely state-restricted, and where these restrictions are maintained by religious leaders and local patrols, only serve to heighten the social, economic, and political control over women's lives and freedoms that enable VAW to occur. As Ferreira and Buttell (p. 136) explain in this issue of *AJPH*, VAW is "both sanctioned and part of the socialization process" for women. The perpetuation of these discriminatory norms combined with the absence of laws and ineffective or lack of intervention or legal response to VAW will only further the endemic nature of this crisis.

PREVENTING VIOLENCE AGAINST WOMEN

The control over women's lives and freedoms that VAW exerts takes many forms—all of which jeopardize the health and safety of women, families, and society. VAW is inextricably linked to worse mental health (e.g., increased depression, anxiety, suicidality), sexual and reproductive health (e.g., increased sexually transmitted infections including HIV, unintended pregnancies), maternal and child health (e.g., increased maternal, infant, and child mortality, decreased pre- and postnatal care), and physical health (e.g., increased injury, food insecurity). Undoing these harms will require multilevel approaches that dismantle the systems and structures that perpetuate control over women's lives and freedoms.

To this point, Alang and Blackstock (p. 194) provide a timely and necessary framework grounded in the principle of health justice that may provide a basis for considering the current systems and structures that sustain VAW. Most importantly, this framework may be particularly germane to preventing VAW as it is driven by the need to enact and implement policies and practices that redistribute power and liberate communities historically disadvantaged by disenfranchisement. Although Alang and Blackstock present the framework specifically in terms mitigating the harms of the COVID-19 pandemic and the HIV epidemic, one can see how this action framework may be applied to undoing the structures and social systems that enable VAW to occur. Furthermore, by grounding the framework's five recommendations in community action and community-based organization, this framework recognizes that we need to simultaneously endeavor to change cultural and societal norms as well as the structures, systems, institutions, laws, and policies that support and enable VAW to be acceptable.

One example of community- and institutional-level action that has immense potential to positively impact responses to VAW is in addressing police response to VAW. A recent report by UN Women titled "Handbook on Gender-Responsive Police Services for Women and Girls Subject to Violence" (https://bit.ly/3AhMDDp) provides a comprehensive set of gender-responsive training guidelines and materials specifically for law enforcement offers. Similarly, in the United States, the International Association of Chiefs of Police has developed a series of materials, resources, and policy recommendations to guide law enforcement officials in responding effectively to VAW (https://bit.ly/2F9ova7).

Changing cultural and societal norms in addition to changing the way police and policing policy are set up to address VAW are two critically needed actions. But equally necessary are efforts to reduce inequalities in the conditions of daily life—ensuring access to adequate and comparable education for all girls and boys, providing equal employment opportunities and job security, reducing food insecurity, and ensuring access to safe and affordable housing. Finally, ensuring health care access that is survivor-centered and enacting laws that support gender equality are the commitments we need across the world to dismantle the structures that underpin acceptance and perpetuation of VAW. In so doing, we will work toward a health justice goal that reaffirms our commitment to women, life, and freedom. AJPH

CORRESPONDENCE

Correspondence should be sent to Farzana Kapadia, PhD, MPH, New York University, School of Global Public Health, 708 Broadway, Room 729, New York, NY 10003 (e-mail: farzana.kapadia@nyu.edu). Reprints can be ordered at https://ajph.org by clicking the "Reprints" link.

PUBLICATION INFORMATION

Full Citation: Kapadia F. Women, life, freedom: a public health of consequence, February 2023. *Am J Public Health*. 2023;113(2):144–145.

Acceptance Date: November 20, 2022.

DOI: https://doi.org/10.2105/AJPH.2022.307186

CONFLICTS OF INTEREST

The author has no conflicts of interest to disclose.

Peace Beyond the Binary: A Creative Intersectional Perspective on Global Forced Displacement

Alli Gillespie, MSW, MPH

ABOUT THE AUTHOR

Alli Gillespie is with the Brown School at Washington University, St Louis, MO.

See also Awor, p. 158, Blum, p. 155, McCullers, p. 149, Vahedi et al., p. 132, and Zimmerman, p. 152.

When I saw a touring version of the musical *Rent* as a 12-year-old, I was enthralled by the characters' fluid, complex identities—and their deep, tender care for one another—as they experienced housing eviction alongside HIV/AIDS illness and death. *Rent* first sparked my curiosity about the intersectional factors that underscore peoples' experiences of forced displacement and shape their resilience.

The main characters respond to the mass eviction of their unhoused neighbors by planning a solidarity-building protest and public performance, which their landlord requests that they cancel to keep the peace in exchange for free housing. They refuse to accept "peace" for their own well-being if it means status-quo violence for others in their community. In a defiant celebration of their queer subculture at the end of the first act, the lead character exclaims: "the opposite of war isn't peace—it's creation!"[1] This lyrical moment spotlights how peace cannot be a crucial determinant of health and well-being if underlying systems of power remain the same; when addressing forced displacement on a global scale, public health responses must instead prioritize dismantling binary social constructs and intentionally creating inclusive care systems.

THE ROLE OF BINARIES IN VIOLENCE AND DISPLACEMENT

Now, as a queer person and a public health student focused on humanitarian contexts and forced migration, I am acutely aware of how the themes of *Rent* continue to resonate in 2022. The global COVID-19 pandemic has intensified existing cycles of violence and displacement generated by structural inequality, poverty, the climate crisis, and political instability.[2,3] These systems operate through divisive, binary social categories—rich and poor, woman and man, Black and White, perpetrator and victim, citizen and foreigner—making people at the intersection of marginalized identity dimensions increasingly vulnerable to violence and forced migration within and across societies.[4] Binary frameworks also determine which displaced populations receive refugee designation and, thus, protection. In this way, "refugee crises" are produced, as nation-states socially construct who is a "deserving [versus] undeserving victim of violence" on one side of a border versus another.[5(p5)] More than ever, public health practitioners must reflect on whether the structures of our programs, our policies, our research, and our organizations actually reproduce, rather than challenge, the binary constructs that perpetuate the cycles of violence we aim to disrupt.

Across interventions to address displacement, the reproduction of binary constructs may seem logical and useful. For example, conceptualizing gender as a binary can allow researchers to statistically analyze and confirm the heightened prevalence of violence victimization among refugee women versus refugee men, and practitioners can address this disparity by implementing women-targeted programming. Binary distinctions can also help a public health practitioner confirm whether a gender-based violence survivor has refugee status and, thus, whether they can legally access support services within certain borders.

However, by relying on binary constructs to inform such a response, researchers and practitioners exclude the complex needs of displaced populations who transcend socially constructed categories in terms of migrant status, gender, race, age group, and a range of other identity dimensions. What if an internally displaced person has an acute need for gender-based violence services and they are intersex, or transgender, or have a disability that prevents them from attending in-person services? All of these individuals may fall outside the target population of many programs as they are currently designed.

Evidence shows that lesbian, gay, bisexual, transgender, queer, or questioning plus (LGBTQ+ or queer) refugees do often face complex barriers to inclusion across contexts because of their intersectional identity dimensions. In addition to their liminal status between citizen and noncitizen, queer refugees must navigate how others will treat them from context to context based on their gender expression and sexual orientation, which can limit their access to resources for health and well-being.

A study of transgender asylum seekers in Mexico found that they experienced discrimination in education and employment based on their evolving gender identities, violence from both their families and state officials, and adverse mental health outcomes.[6] In another study, LGBTQ+ refugees and asylees living in a range of contexts in the United States and Canada reported widespread experiences of violence and a lack of support resources and protection across institutional levels and locations.[7] These studies highlight how refugees who transcend binary constructs face violence and displacement not just from their communities but also from a migrant protection apparatus designed for refugees whose identities are assumed to fit neatly into predetermined boxes.

DECONSTRUCTING BINARY SYSTEMS WITH CREATIVE INTERSECTIONALITY

Applying the lens of intersectionality is crucial for understanding the link between binary constructs and the perpetuation of displacement. Kimberlé Crenshaw's original use of the framework explored how binary conceptions of gender and race in the US legal system produced differential access to systems of justice for women who had experienced violence; the structural separation of racial discrimination and gender discrimination privileged White women's and Black men's experiences and obscured the cross-cutting effects of gender and race for Black women.[8] In seeking to address forced displacement, I argue that we must incorporate an expanded version of intersectionality—what I call "creative intersectionality"—that explores how global systems of power relate to and shape one another, recognizes that identity dimensions are not dichotomous nor essential but are developed by translocational experiences and sociocultural contexts, and prioritizes critical action to deconstruct binaries in favor of new systems for collective well-being.[9,10]

For example, using creative intersectionality as a lens to understand and ultimately address forced displacement requires that we examine all forms of binary constructs, and not just those imposed on an individual's identity dimensions. Dubal et al. posit that we must move beyond analyzing the social determinants of health (such as gender, race, and class) to confront "infrastructural determinants of health" such as nation-state borders. As binary constructs of "in" versus "out," borders provide an illusion of peace among their elite while simultaneously displacing people and "distinguishing who does and does not have the right to access care."[11]

Applying creative intersectionality unveils this illusion and invites us to dig deeper into why those borders exist in the first place. Creative intersectionality as a perspective for addressing forced displacement thus falls under the broader strategy of decolonization or "dismantling the [violent] legacy of formal colonialism and imagining its replacement."[9(p109)] It is also guided by the leadership of Indigenous resurgence scholars such as Leanne Betasamosake Simpson, who avows that "we can't have resurgence without centering gender and queerness, and creating alternative systems of accountability for sexual and gender violence."[12(p30)]

The opposite of war isn't peace. It's creation. Creation can mean uplifting participatory, qualitative research methods wherein people can construct their lived experiences apart from the fixed categories assigned to them. It can mean including more gender options in a survey than "man or woman." Creation can include legitimizing chosen families and other kinship structures rather than privileging biological nuclear families. It can mean building local mutual aid networks for anyone who requests resources and support rather than limiting service eligibility based on identity requirements. Creation is making intentional space for and amplifying the leadership of those not represented by dichotomous categorizations or the systems of power maintained by binaries and borders. Creation is bolstering indigenous peoples' power with collective land and resources. The current moment of climate and health crises is a crucial one. If the field of public health wants to reduce forced displacement and to promote global peace as a determinant of health and well-being, we must use creative intersectionality to construct inclusive care systems within and across contexts. AJPH

CORRESPONDENCE

Correspondence should be sent to Alli Gillespie, Washington University in St Louis, 1 Brookings Dr, St Louis, MO 63130 (e-mail: a.gillespie@wustl.edu). Reprints can be ordered at https://ajph.org by clicking the "Reprints" link.

PUBLICATION INFORMATION

Full Citation: Gillespie A. Peace beyond the binary: a creative intersectional perspective on global forced displacement. *Am J Public Health*. 2023; 113(2):146–148.

Acceptance Date: November 16, 2022.

DOI: https://doi.org/10.2105/AJPH.2022.307177

ACKNOWLEDGMENTS

The author would like to thank Ilana Seff, DrPH, for the mentorship that she provided as an MPH practicum field instructor during the drafting of this editorial.

CONFLICTS OF INTEREST

The author has no conflicts of interest to disclose.

REFERENCES

1. Original Broadway Cast Recording. *La Vie Bohème From Rent*. DreamWorks; 1996.
2. Kim J, Rivas Mor Mur MJ, Dahlgren E, Cruz Valladares R. The impact of COVID-19 on forced displacement: addressing the challenges and harnessing the opportunities of a crisis. Reference paper for the 70th Anniversary of the 1951 Refugee Convention. United Nations High Commissioner for Refugees. 2021. Available at: https://www.unhcr.org/people-forced-to-flee-book/wp-content/uploads/sites/137/2021/10/Julie-Kim-et-al_The-Impact-of-COVID-19-on-Forced-Displacement.pdf. Accessed November 28, 2022.
3. Gillespie A, Seff I, Caron C, et al. "The pandemic made us stop and think about who we are and what we want": using intersectionality to understand migrant and refugee women's experiences of gender-based violence during COVID-19. *BMC Public Health*. 2022;22(1):1469. https://doi.org/10.1186/s12889-022-13866-7
4. Shelton J, Dodd SJ. Binary thinking and the limiting of human potential. *Public Integr*. 2021;23(6):624–635. https://doi.org/10.1080/10999922.2021.1988405
5. Carastathis A, Kouri-Towe N, Mahrouse G, Whitley L. Introduction. *Refuge*. 2018;34(1):3–15. https://doi.org/10.7202/1050850ar
6. Cheney MK, Gowin MJ, Taylor EL, et al. Living outside the gender box in Mexico: testimony of transgender Mexican asylum seekers. *Am J Public Health*. 2017;107(10):1646–1652. https://doi.org/10.2105/AJPH.2017.303961
7. Alessi EJ, Kahn S, Chatterji S. "The darkest times of my life": recollections of child abuse among forced migrants persecuted because of their sexual orientation and gender identity. *Child Abuse Negl*. 2016;51:93–105. https://doi.org/10.1016/j.chiabu.2015.10.030
8. Crenshaw K. Mapping the margins: intersectionality, identity politics, and violence against women of color. *Stanford Law Rev*. 1991;43(6):1241–1299. https://doi.org/10.2307/1229039
9. Collins PH. *Intersectionality as Critical Social Theory*. Durham, NC: Duke University Press; 2019. https://doi.org/10.1215/9781478007098
10. Anthias F. Transnational mobilities, migration research and intersectionality: towards a translocational frame. *Nord J Migr Res*. 2012;2(2):102. https://doi.org/10.2478/v10202-011-0032-y
11. Dubal SB, Samra SS, Janeway HH. Beyond border health: infrastructural violence and the health of border abolition. *Soc Sci Med*. 2021;279:113967. https://doi.org/10.1016/j.socscimed.2021.113967
12. Simpson LB. Indigenous resurgence and co-resistance. *Critical Ethnic Studies*. 2016;2(2):19–34. https://doi.org/10.5749/jcritethnstud.2.2.0019

The Peace Exchange: Physical and Psychological Sacrifices of Military Personnel From Historically Marginalized Backgrounds

Asli McCullers, BS

ABOUT THE AUTHOR

Asli McCullers is with the College of Health Sciences, University of Delaware, Newark, DE.

See also Awor, p. 158, Blum, p. 155, Gillespie, p. 146, Vahedi et al., p. 132, and Zimmerman, p. 152.

The physical and psychological well-being of both active-duty military personnel and military veterans in the United States remains a critical topic in public health research and advocacy. Nearly one in four active-duty military and military veterans report having some form of mental illness, with over 6000 military suicides occurring annually.[1,2] In our efforts as public health professionals, there should remain space to amplify the stories that describe the experiences of the many military personnel with historically marginalized backgrounds. Such personnel include those who represent racial and ethnic minorities, low-income backgrounds, sexual and gender minorities, and an array of other systemically oppressed identities. Underdiscussed to date are frameworks that express the pursuit of population-level peace and safety serving dually as a motivator for enlisting in military service and, unfortunately, in turn operating as a determinant of poor health outcomes among military personnel, especially those of marginalized backgrounds. The aim of this brief editorial is to further strengthen the ongoing conversation regarding how to improve the health of marginalized military personnel who sacrifice their personal welfare to maintain peace in a country where they have historically been oppressed.

FINDING PURPOSE IN PEACE: MOTIVATIONS FOR ENLISTING

Military personnel are often recruited into service with the motivation of serving a role in maintaining peace and safety in the United States. Core to military training is the goal of protecting communities from external threats. In a 2018 RAND Corporation study, more than one-fourth of new military recruits reported that their "call to serve" was a strong motivating factor for their enlistments.[3] To perhaps an equal or greater degree of motivation to enlist are the financial and occupational benefits.[3] The intersection of these two motivations leads to many military recruits being people of color from poor or vulnerable communities. African American men, for example, are overrepresented in the military in comparison with African American men in the civilian labor force by a ratio of 2:1.[4] My parents, who are both military veterans, have beginnings that mirror these statistics. My mother and father hail from extremely humble, Deep South backgrounds, representing rural African American communities in Alabama and North Carolina, respectively. They reflect often on how, growing up, their families engaged in a 20th-century form of sharecropping for income. As children, they would spend summers working in the fields, experiencing the firsthand consequences of systemic oppression, financial disenfranchisement, and structural racism. When my parents decided to enlist in the military in the 1980s, it provided them with opportunities to bring protection, progression, and *peace* back home to their communities, as well as financial support. Even now, this is the story of many low-income people of color considering joining the military—a way out and a way up.

Although the intent of many military recruits is to gain opportunity and stability while protecting and serving their communities, the price that many pay expands beyond their wildest fears. Post-traumatic stress disorder, depression, and chronic illness are just the tip of the iceberg of conditions that impact military personnel and veterans vastly. Once young soldiers with the hope of bringing protection, progress, and peace to their communities, my

AJPH February 2023, Vol 113, No. 2

parents are now a part of the roughly 3.5 million veterans that are both chronically ill and disabled.[5] Outwardly, many veterans express pride and reflect on their service with valor. But behind the "thank you for your service" comments and the free meal on Veterans Day is the endurance of unthinkable suffering that consumes the mental and physical peace of millions of veterans annually. The illusion of peace as a population-level determinant of health comes at the grim expense of peace and well-being on an individual level for military veterans.

AT A GLANCE: WHAT WE'RE LEARNING AND WHAT WE CAN DO

Reimagining peace as both a population- and individual-level determinant of health should be considered through the lens of military personnel. Specifically, space should exist to consider what this means for military personnel of diverse backgrounds. Below are three driving points that may be helpful in framing these conversations:

1. *Unpacking the illusion of peace*: From the COVID-19 pandemic to the climax of the Black Lives Matter movement, the sociopolitical chaos that has defined the past two years has evidenced our country's imperative need to look inward at our internal points of instability. Spanning the lives of all living generations, the US military has largely been viewed as among the most powerful forces of defense in the world and a beacon of peacekeeping for Americans. However, as a nation, we are beginning to address the incredibly dark US history of global imperialism, colonization, and violence more openly against recovering nations of color and the way these harmful practices are often associated with the armed forces.[6] Masked by obligatory patriotism and nationalism, "the illusion of peace" within the United States has become markedly apparent. We have a long way to go before our national defense truly functions as a source of population-level peace maintenance that centers on social justice domestically and globally.
2. *Health equity through a military lens*: Unraveling how the illusion of peace is structurally built into the armed forces aids our ability to recognize how ever-present inequity is within the military. The strength of the US military has been built largely on the backs of vulnerable soldiers from low-income, marginalized communities. The health equity implications of this are widespread. Men and women who are African American, Hispanic, and of other races report worse self-rated health, greater Veterans Affairs healthcare use, and more combat exposure than their White counterparts.[7] Continued efforts to address how health inequity manifests in military contexts is critical to ensuring that minoritized personnel will not face worse health outcomes.
3. *Advocacy and action*: Work to improve the lives of military personnel of diverse backgrounds must extend beyond "conversations and commentaries" such as this one. Organizations such as Minority Veterans of America, American Latino Veterans Association, National Association for Black Veterans, and many others have made strides in creating justice-oriented initiatives that make health equity actionable for veterans. Such initiatives include job placement assistance and support navigating Veterans Affairs claims and mental health resources. In addition, further expansion into and investment in public service programs such as AmeriCorps could provide alternative options for young people looking to engage in peacekeeping work.

CONCLUSION

The physical and mental health sacrifices that military personnel make by joining the service speak to a greater picture that illustrates how peace and safety, which should both stand as fundamental rights for all, are far from being well embedded in the culture of the United States. On the pathway to attaining population-level stability and peace, military personnel sacrifice peace within their own minds and bodies. This is a schismatic phenomenon and public health crisis that must not persist further. True peace will hopefully someday come at no cost to anyone, regardless of their occupational choices, upbringing, or background. A military infrastructure that decenters violence and global domination and instead centers on justice for all, authentically, should define the future of peacekeeping for the next generation. AJPH

CORRESPONDENCE

Correspondence should be sent to Asli McCullers, 100 Discovery Boulevard, Newark, DE 19711 (email: amccul@udel.edu). Reprints can be ordered at http://www.ajph.org by clicking the "Reprints" link.

PUBLICATION INFORMATION

Full Citation: McCullers A. The peace exchange: physical and psychological sacrifices of military personnel from historically marginalized backgrounds. *Am J Public Health*. 2023;113(2):149–151.

Acceptance Date: November 16, 2022.
DOI: https://doi.org/10.2105/AJPH.2022.307178

ACKNOWLEDGMENTS

The author acknowledges her parents, Gregory and Shelia McCullers, for their service in the United States Army and for being the inspiration for this work.

CONFLICTS OF INTEREST

The author has no conflicts of interest to disclose.

REFERENCES

1. National Alliance on Mental Illness. Veterans & Active Duty. Available at: https://www.nami.org/Your-Journey/Veterans-Active-Duty. Accessed July 27, 2022.
2. Inoue C, Shawler E, Jordan CH, Jackson CA. Veteran and military mental health issues. In: *StatPearls*. Treasure Island, FL: StatPearls Publishing; May 23, 2022.
3. Helmus TC, Zimmerman SR, Posard MN, Wheeler JL, Stroud Q, Harrell MC. *Life as a Private: A Study of the Motivations and Experiences of Junior Enlisted Personnel in the US Army*. Santa Monica, CA: RAND Corporation; 2018.
4. Reeves RV, Nzau S. Black Americans are much more likely to serve the nation, in military and civilian roles. Brookings. Published August 27, 2020. Available at: https://www.brookings.edu/blog/up-front/2020/08/27/black-americans-are-much-more-likely-to-serve-the-nation-in-military-and-civilian-roles/. Accessed July 27, 2022.
5. ADA National Network. Employment Data for Veterans With Disabilities. Published 2017. Available at: https://adata.org/factsheet/employment-data-veterans-disabilities#:~:text=Nearly%20a%20third%20(29.6%25%2C,report%20only%20a%20SC%20disability. Accessed July 27, 2022.
6. Haass RN. The use and abuse of military force. Brookings. Published November 1, 1999. Available at: https://www.brookings.edu/research/the-use-and-abuse-of-military-force/. Accessed July 27, 2022.
7. Ward RE, Nguyen XT, Li Y, et al. Racial and ethnic disparities in US veteran health characteristics. Int J Environ Res Public Health. 2021;18(5):2411.

Honoring Dignity in Violent Times

Brett Zimmerman, BA

ABOUT THE AUTHOR

Brett Zimmerman is a Master of Public Health student, Simmons University, Boston, MA.

See also Awor, p. 158, Blum, p. 155, Gillespie, p. 146, McCullers, p. 149, and Vahedi et al., p. 132.

The night had been busy, and stabbing calls usually sounded much worse over dispatch than the reality on-scene. It was easy to keep my eyes closed in the back of the fire engine as we rumbled to the call. The blue light of police cars illuminated the open front door. I got to her first, following a trail of blood down the narrow hallway to a back bedroom. A police officer knelt, holding pressure on her neck, his face white. Her eyes seemed ready to leap from her face, her brown skin tinged gray. A faint five o'clock shadow threatened the edges of her mouth. Opening the medical kit, I retrieved a trauma pad to slide under the officer's gloved hands.

As we worked, she mouthed, sometimes rasped, for help. Her hands grasped at shirts, the wall, our hands, finally, fiercely, clutching my right hand. My partners worked a lifting tarp under her, asking if we were ready to roll him. The police officer, hands still pressed to her neck, quickly corrected them: "Her. She uses 'her.'"

Three of us carried her down the hallway, to the waiting ambulance, the police officer still holding pressure. The paramedics met us with the gurney. As we slid her onto the stretcher, they asked how he had been stabbed. Again, the officer corrected, "She uses 'she.'" The lead medic snorted, shook his head, and grunted a "whatever."

We rolled the gurney to the back of the ambulance as he rested two fingers lightly on the frame. I took the police officer's place at her neck, climbing inside before the back doors banged shut.

INCREASING VIOLENCE TARGETING TRANSGENDER COMMUNITIES

This happened in 2018, a year after a different Portland, Oregon, stabbing. A White supremacist stabbed three passengers in the neck on a commuter train. They had intervened in his racist rant directed at two young passengers of color. One survived. Violence against systematically marginalized groups is on the rise,[1] coalescing into domestic instability fueled by dehumanizing political rhetoric and targeted legislation that limits access to voting and gender-affirming and reproductive health care. There are moments of desperation when defending the dignity of a dying person may be the only way to access our interconnected humanity. But, it is not enough. Indifference to violence intended to dehumanize must be met with collective urgency to challenge structural violence[2] with structural protections that affirm the inherent dignity that underpins our human rights.

Violence is concentrated in the intersections of oppressed identities.[3] The year 2021 was the deadliest year on record for transgender people in America.[4] Black transgender women accounted for two thirds of known victims of fatal violence against transgender people since 2013.[4] In 2019, the American Medical Association declared an epidemic of antitransgender violence, especially against Black transgender women.[5] Increasing threats of physical violence are paralleled by the record-setting introduction of 155 state-level antitrans bills by October 2022.[6] This legislation seeks to codify trans people out of existence by criminalizing access to gender-affirming care, restricting participation in organized sports, implementing "bathroom bills," and prohibiting the correction of identification documents.[6] Only 16 states have banned "gay/trans panic" legal defense strategies that allow perpetrators of violence to blame their actions on their victim's gender or sexuality.[7]

A healthy democracy demands equal access and full participation. Antitrans structural and sectarian violence restricts the ability of transgender people, especially Black trans women, to fully participate in society. The othering implicit in antitrans legislation kindles violence out of entitlement to civic participation and state protection for some, but not for all. Self-determination and bodily autonomy are rights, not privileges. Laws and policies that suggest otherwise create distinctions between groups that are antithetical to the social cohesion instrumental to peaceful democracy.

An increasingly bold and extreme sect of the far right seeks to further restrict the rights of systematically minoritized groups while simultaneously challenging the legitimacy of our democracy. The belief that the rules do not apply evenly, and to everyone, was echoed in the January 6th rallying cry to "take back *our* country." It is evident

AJPH February 2023, Vol 113, No. 2

in the violent protests against the perceived violation of bodily autonomy via mask mandates while the American Medical Association and pediatric care organizations are imploring the Justice Department to investigate threats of violence against providers and families of children seeking gender-affirming care.[8] Fear of dispossession radicalizes rhetoric into violence. Ijeoma Oluo describes the "desperation, disappointment, despair, and rage"[9] that accompanies fear of perceived irrelevance. An increase in interpersonal violence against trans people is augmented by organized extremist violence at Pride parades and drag queen story hours. A sense of entitlement to the benefits of society, while simultaneously denying them to others, is consistent with the realities of the history of our nation but not the spirit of the democratic experiment.

DIGNITY AS THE BEDROCK FOR STRUCTURAL CHANGE

Structural violence requires structural solutions. Affirming inherent human dignity is fundamental but, on its own, is not enough. Creating refuges for transgender people to access care, or exist without fear of violence, is critical. And still not enough. As public health professionals, we are asked to look to root causes to find solutions for ill health. Our collective ill health is in the weakness of our legislative bodies to draft unwavering protections of the right to self-determination for all people. Only 54% of lesbian, gay, bisexual, transgender, queer plus (LGBTQ+) people live in a state where their gender identity is protected under hate crime laws.[10] In an increasingly sectarian environment, the states have proven they are not honest protectors of human rights, and federal legislation is needed to protect the rights to bodily autonomy and self-determination. Furthermore, there must be federal action to improve consistency and effectiveness in existing hate crime legislation that accounts for motivations in increasing antitrans violence.

In a democracy, the power of our institutions derives from civic participation. Though it is necessary to establish political power to restore the capacities limited by violence, this same violence isolates the communities it targets. Healthy People 2030 lists "social cohesion" under social and community determinants of health.[11] This collective efficacy hinges on community trust and solidarity, guiding community members to follow social norms that result in lower rates of neighborhood violence and improved health.[11] As trust builds social cohesion, it, in turn, highlights our interdependence. In this interdependence is our collective fate as a democracy. Social cohesion reveals our shared liberation from structures that oppress us all when they oppress any of us.

Former United Nations Secretary General Ban Ki-moon declared peace dependent on the recognition of human "dignity, rights and capacities" for all people.[12] Our ability to create fully democratic institutions relies on our collective capacity that emerges from understanding that we are all diminished until we are all free. The trust required to build social cohesion begins with believing in each other's right to dignity. In the face of growing structural violence, concern over dignity may seem meek. But honoring dignity is not nothing. In fact, it could be everything. Allowing someone their full self in turn allows us our full selves. We dignify ourselves when we dignify others. AJPH

CORRESPONDENCE

Correspondence should be sent to Brett Zimmerman, Simmons University, 300 The Fenway, Public Health Department, Room C320H, Boston, MA 02115 (e-mail: brett.zimmerman@gmail.com). Reprints can be ordered at https://ajph.org by clicking the "Reprints" link.

PUBLICATION INFORMATION

Full Citation: Zimmerman B. Honoring dignity in violent times. *Am J Public Health*. 2023;113(2): 152–154.

Acceptance Date: November 16, 2022.

DOI: https://doi.org/10.2105/AJPH.2022.307180

CONFLICTS OF INTEREST

The author has no conflicts of interest to disclose.

REFERENCES

1. Farivar M. US hate crimes rise during first half of 2022. *Voice of America News.* August 23, 2002. Available at: https://www.voanews.com/a/us-hate-crimes-rise-during-first-half-of-2022-/6713791.html. Accessed November 4, 2022.
2. Farmer PE, Nizeye B, Stulac S, Keshavjee S. Structural violence and clinical medicine. *PLoS Med.* 2006;3(10):e449. https://doi.org/10.1371/journal.pmed.0030449
3. Crenshaw K. The urgency of intersectionality. TED Talk. 2016. Available at: https://www.youtube.com/watch?v=7rsJcj6sbQw. Accessed December 1, 2022.
4. Human Rights Campaign. An epidemic of violence 2021. Available at: https://reports.hrc.org/an-epidemic-of-violence-fatal-violence-against-transgender-and-gender-non-confirming-people-in-the-united-states-in-2021#. Accessed November 4, 2022.
5. American Medical Association. AMA adopts new polices on first day of voting at 2019 Annual Meeting. June 10, 2019. Available at: https://www.ama-assn.org/press-center/press-releases/ama-adopts-new-policies-first-day-voting-2019-annual-meeting. Accessed July 27, 2022.
6. Branigan A, Kirkpatrick N. Anti-transgender laws are on the rise. *Washington Post.* October 14, 2022. Available at: https://www.washingtonpost.com/lifestyle/2022/10/14/anti-trans-bills. Accessed November 4, 2022.
7. The LGBTQ+ Bar. LGBTQ+ "panic" defense. Available at: https://lgbtqbar.org/programs/advocacy/gay-trans-panic-defense. Accessed July 27, 2022.
8. Greenesmith H. Violence against transgender people is on the rise, stopping it requires a holistic solution. Just Security. October 18, 2022. Available at: https://www.justsecurity.org/83597/violence-against-transgender-people-is-on-the-rise-stopping-it-requires-a-holistic-solution. Accessed November 4, 2022.
9. Mosley T, Hagan A. Author Ijeoma Oluo's "Mediocre" confronts White male power in America. WBUR. Here & Now; December 16, 2020. Available at: https://www.wbur.org/hereandnow/2020/12/16/ijeoma-oluo-mediocre-book. Accessed July 27, 2022.

10. Movement Advancement Project. Policy spotlight: hate crime laws. Available at: https://www.lgbtmap.org/2021-report-hate-crimes. Accessed November 4, 2022.
11. Healthy People 2030. Social cohesion. Office of Disease Prevention and Health Promotion, Department of Health and Human Services. Available at: https://health.gov/healthypeople/priority-areas/social-determinants-health/literature-summaries/social-cohesion. Accessed July 27, 2022.
12. Peace means dignity, well-being for all, not just absence of war. *UN News*. September 9, 2014. Available at: https://news.un.org/en/story/2014/09/476992-peace-means-dignity-well-being-all-not-just-absence-war-un-officials. Accessed July 27, 2022.

Forgotten People in Forgotten Places: The Uncounted Costs of Conflict

Alexander J. Blum, MPH

ABOUT THE AUTHOR

Alexander J. Blum is an MD candidate (class of 2023) at the Johns Hopkins University School of Medicine, Baltimore, MD.

See also Awor, p. 158, Gillespie, p. 146, McCullers, p. 149, Vahedi et al, p. 132, and Zimmerman, p. 152.

"Kaka, please help." Wincing as he described the pain in his leg, the 65-year-old Burundian patient sat down in the clinic. Expressing gratitude—and a palpable hope that medical care could help him—Emmanuel (patient's name and identifying information changed to protect privacy) shared more about the tortuous series of events that precipitated him seeking care at the Tanzania Red Cross health center in Nyarugusu refugee camp in western Tanzania in April 2022. I was there as a student with several physicians from my medical school as we participated in clinical care and bidirectional learning as part of a long-standing relationship with the Tanzania Red Cross Society.

Emmanuel's gaze caught my own. As we witnessed one another for a prolonged moment, I thought about how different our lives had been and the profound injustice of our disparate circumstances.

A longtime refugee originally from Burundi, Emmanuel shared that more than 10 years before, he began to have trouble urinating. As the problem worsened, he sought help from clinicians in Nyarugusu refugee camp. The doctors suspected that he had an enlarged prostate and added him to a list of referral patients who would need more advanced work-up—and possibly intervention—from facilities outside the camp. As is the case in most refugee camps across the world, the referral process is often lengthy and unpredictable, with a committee meeting once monthly to discuss patients for possible referral.[1] Seeking treatment or referral can be an especially difficult ordeal for elderly patients, as a majority of resources in humanitarian settings are often directed toward younger women and children.[2]

Frustrated by the process and desperate for relief, Emmanuel resolved to take matters into his own hands. Because he was a refugee, it was illegal for him to leave the camp without permission.[1] However, the camp's borders were relatively fluid, and there were no strict boundaries or checkpoints to prevent people from leaving the camp. Spending a significant sum of his family's savings and assuming great personal risk by leaving the camp to cross an international border, Emmanuel traveled to Burundi and paid out of pocket for a surgery to remove his prostate. Although his urinary symptoms improved, the surgery likely damaged a nerve, which left him with chronic, painful neuropathy. He has been debilitated by the pain ever since but is unable to seek follow-up care with his surgeon in Burundi given the prohibitive cost and risks of traveling.

Tracing the roots of Emmanuel's story reveals the profoundly dysfunctional and fundamentally unjust nature of dramatically underresourced health systems that are tasked with providing care to refugee populations across the globe. I do not share Emmanuel's story to blame clinicians or public health practitioners who do valiant work caring for refugee populations every day. Rather, I hope to demonstrate the challenges these individuals face by working in underfunded and perpetually overburdened systems.[3]

Above all, Emmanuel's experience shows how individuals displaced by conflict and violence continue to bear the burdens of war decades later. The longterm morbidity and mortality of displaced populations are rarely taken into account when reporting the human costs of a conflict, but their continued suffering is both real and unjust. By a mere accident of birth, Emmanuel and nearly one billion other migrants and refugees across the world find themselves in circumstances plagued by uncertainty, instability, and ceaseless challenges.[4]

Indeed, peace and stability are undeniably necessary (albeit not sufficient) determinants of health. Without these foundations, clinical care is tenuous at best and entirely absent at worst. The collapse of health care in tandem with the dissolution of stability is exemplified in places such as Venezuela and Lebanon,

AJPH February 2023, Vol 113, No. 2

where the undoing of these countries' once stable—even if unjust—political regimes has led to the rapid decline of health care services.[5,6] Without a foundation of stability and peace, clinical management of common conditions such as hypertension, diabetes, and commonplace surgical disease becomes exceedingly challenging. This leaves survivors of conflict suffering from an overwhelming burden of readily preventable and treatable morbidity. For those with more complicated conditions, such as cancer, proper work-up and adequate treatment with long-term surveillance is nonexistent.

In refugee camp settings designed to handle only basic medical conditions on a temporary basis—and often with an emphasis on maternal and child health—providing quality medical and surgical care for an elderly patient like Emmanuel is exceedingly challenging. Systems of care to adequately address many conditions requiring long-term treatment (e.g., hypertension, diabetes, tuberculosis) have never materialized. Entire populations are left at the mercy of fragile systems that were designed to triage and stabilize, not to treat long term. Despite this, most refugee camps become long-term settlements, and it is rare for political processes to ethically resettle people expeditiously. Indeed, the World Health Organization (WHO) recently released its first ever report on refugees and migrants.[4] These populations' absence in global surveys and health data "make them almost invisible in the design of health systems and services," noted the WHO director general Tedros Adhanom Ghebreyesus.[7]

Despite formally enshrined doctrines proclaiming health as a human right,[8,9] migrants and refugees are rarely afforded access to high-quality or subspeciality care, which is often deemed too costly or difficult to provide in these settings.[10] Tragically, cost–benefit analyses of medical care in humanitarian settings are often grounded in well-intentioned assessments of currently available resources, although more can and should be done to change this. Discussions of cost effectiveness do little to help patients with active pathologies today: the mother with severe postpartum hemorrhage, the child with leukemia, or the elderly man with an enlarged prostate.

In the absence of care, these individuals—like any of us—may reasonably try to seek treatment elsewhere. For Emmanuel, this entailed spending extensive savings to journey across the border into Burundi, where he received an operation that ultimately left him more impoverished and disabled than he was before seeking care. He has been suffering in Nyarugusu for years. His impoverishment and lack of access to care, which forced him to leave the refugee camp, can ultimately be traced to the conflict in Burundi that displaced him and his family many years ago.

Despite the enormity of the challenges facing migrants and refugees today, meaningful change is well within reach. Investments to strengthen health systems in refugee camp settings should be made in partnership with host communities, which often face similar burdens of poverty and clinical destitution. Instead of being banned from working, refugees should be employed, empowered, and trained to establish health infrastructure in the places where they are to be resettled. No refugee or asylee, many of whom have endured violence and persecution, should be discharged and condemned to a clinical desert.

This is readily doable, and it would not take vast investments to improve the current standard of care in most refugee camp settings. The ordeals endured by patients like Emmanuel demonstrate the human toll shouldered by those continuing to bear the cost of conflict and the absence of peace in their home communities. If we are to truly recognize and ameliorate the suffering of our world's one billion migrants and refugees, we would do well to focus on strengthening health systems with equity and inclusivity as our guiding principles. AJPH

CORRESPONDENCE

Correspondence should be sent to Alexander J. Blum, 1600 McElderry St, Baltimore, MD 21205 (e-mail: ablum16@jhmi.edu). Reprints can be ordered at http://www.ajph.org by clicking the "Reprints" link.

PUBLICATION INFORMATION

Full Citation: Blum AJ. Forgotten people in forgotten places: the uncounted costs of conflict. *Am J Public Health*. 2023;113(2):155–157.

Acceptance Date: November 16, 2022.

DOI: https://doi.org/10.2105/AJPH.2022.307179

ACKNOWLEDGMENTS

A. J. Blum's travel to Tanzania in March–April 2022 was supported by Balch Grant Award funding from the Department of Surgery, Johns Hopkins Hospital.

I express my special gratitude to the Tanzanian, Congolese, and Burundian health care workers who dedicate their lives to caring for vulnerable communities.

CONFLICTS OF INTEREST

The author has no conflicts of interest to report.

REFERENCES

1. Enumah ZO. Therapeutic citizens or therapeutic refugees? An examination of triage, refugeehood, and referral health care in Tanzania. *Soc Sci Med*. 2022;298:114837. https://doi.org/10.1016/j.socscimed.2022.114837
2. Robinson A, Marella M, Logam L. Gap analysis on the inclusion of people with disability and older people in humanitarian response. August 7, 2020. Available at: https://www.elrha.org/researchdatabase/gap-analysis-humanitarian-inclusion-disabilities-older-people-literature-review. Accessed November 28, 2022.
3. Spiegel PB. The humanitarian system is not just broke, but broken: recommendations for future humanitarian action. *Lancet*. [Online ahead of print June 7, 2017]. https://doi.org/10.1016/S0140-6736(17)31278-3

4. World Health Organization. World report on the health of refugees and migrants: summary. July 20, 2022. Available at: https://www.who.int/publications/i/item/9789240054462. Accessed November 28, 2022.
5. Hubbard B. Collapse: inside Lebanon's worst economic meltdown in more than a century. *New York Times*. August 4, 2021. Available at: https://www.nytimes.com/2021/08/04/world/lebanon-crisis.html. Accessed July 20, 2022.
6. Lancet. The collapse of the Venezuelan health system. *Lancet*. 2018;391(10128):1331. https://doi.org/10.1016/S0140-6736(16)00277-4
7. Schlein L. WHO: millions of refugees, migrants suffer ill health for lack of care. July 20 2022. Available at: https://www.voanews.com/a/who-millions-of-refugees-migrants-suffer-ill-health-for-lack-of-care/6666920.html. Accessed July 21, 2022.
8. UN General Assembly. Convention relating to the status of refugees, 28 July 1951, United Nations. Treaty Series, vol. 189, p. 137. Available at: https://www.refworld.org/docid/3be01b964.html. Accessed July 20, 2022.
9. UN General Assembly. Transforming our world: the 2030 Agenda for Sustainable Development, 21 October 2015, A/RES/70/1. Available at: https://www.refworld.org/docid/57b6e3e44.html. Accessed July 20, 2022.
10. Mateen FJ, Spiegel PB. How Should relief organizations fund care of patient-asylees who have cancer? *AMA J Ethics*. 2022;24(6):E457–E462. https://doi.org/10.1001/amajethics.2022.457

Pathways to Peace and Public Health Equity Among Women and Children in Conflict Zones: The Case of Northern Uganda

Susan Awor, MPH

ABOUT THE AUTHOR

Susan Awor is an emerging researcher and Global Health Fellow with the School of Public Health, University of California, Berkeley.

See also Blum, p. 155, Gillespie, p. 146, McCullers, p. 149, Vahedi et al., p. 132, and Zimmerman, p. 152.

Peace is one of the major prerequisites for the preservation of health. Without it, basic needs of life such as food, water, and shelter cannot be assured. Historical evidence has linked disease outbreaks to war conditions. In 430 BC, the Plague of Athens was exacerbated by overcrowding during the Peloponnesian War,[1] and poor nutrition in cramped military camps worsened the deadly Spanish flu of 1918.[2]

Although the mortality burden is mostly borne by men, women and children are a soft target in armed conflict because they are more vulnerable to poverty, discrimination, and sexual violence.[3] In countries like Yemen and Syria, persistent conflicts amid deeply ingrained patriarchal ideologies reinforce structural violence, culminating in the torture, rape, and murder of women and girls. Moreover, strict conservatism and attitudes about gender roles restrict them from working, which makes it extremely difficult to afford health care. In Nigeria, the Boko Haram target and enslave schoolgirls as a weapon to wage war against communities. A similar tactic against women and children was used by the Lord's Resistance Army (LRA), as witnessed by the author in her own home area of northern Uganda.

Joseph Kony led the LRA movement in 1986 after Yoweri Museveni's government overthrew the former regime run by an ethnic Acholi from northern Uganda. Kony's self-described motive was the establishment of a theocratic state for the redemption of his people, but he instead victimized them. The author's extended family had a beautiful traditional homestead in Otuke-Lango, bordering the Acholi subregion. Women participated in domestic roles such as cooking, child nurturing, fetching water, planting, and harvesting, while men traded in animal hides and skins. Children enjoyed all forms of creative play, sport, and performing arts. But a village that was relatively peaceful would soon become the target of the LRA. In the late 1990s, surprise attacks began in Lango and went on for more than a decade. Rape, massacres, arson, and mutilation were the order of the day, with women and children abducted as sex slaves and soldiers. One fateful day in June 2000, while digging in Omoro, the author's brother, who was only 11 years old at the time, received a tip-off about a possible rebel invasion. He abandoned his hoe and dared to run but was abducted at the Okuru River, across which he could not swim. The rebels flogged him ruthlessly, then handed him ammunition to join them in carrying out killings. For years he was both a victim and a perpetrator, inflicting grave atrocities against civilians by order of the LRA for his own survival. In December 2004, he escaped captivity during an ambush as the rebels crossed the Ugandan border into South Sudan. He sought safety in an internally displaced people's camp, where he received amnesty; despite rehabilitation, however, the horrors of the LRA war that left thousands of people killed are forever etched in his mind. To this day, he suffers some physical disability and partial hearing loss. The author's broader community grappled with an increased burden of care for orphans, early adolescent pregnancies, incident HIV infections, and loss of livelihood opportunities. Mental health and psychosocial support were neglected and, as of now, many victims have still not healed.

United Nations (UN) Security Council Resolution 1325 on Women, Peace, and Security,[4] adopted in October 2000, proposed a framework to deal with several challenges women face in situations of conflict. Despite their adoption by several countries, there is limited evidence to show that the objectives of such frameworks have been significantly achieved. The author acknowledges the tremendous efforts by the UN, global development actors, and governments championing key interventions toward securing peace and health equity in regions confronted with conflict. In the author's opinion, more effort could be directed toward examining risk factors and harmonizing multilevel approaches to improve mental well-being and prevent recurrence of conflict.

In their article,[5] Link and Phelan invite us to contextualize social conditions as fundamental causes of disease if we are to craft effective interventions to promote population health. In most conflict situations, the intersectionality of gender and low socioeconomic status translates into discrimination and differential access to resources, which serve as upstream factors that place people and communities at risk. By identifying how vulnerable groups become marginalized, and working in partnership with them, stakeholders can establish multilevel interventions to counter the consequences of conflict.

The social-ecological model helps us to better understand drivers of conflict and identify opportunities to intervene at different levels. In the author's community, traditional strategies—such as "*mato oput*,"[6] which involves ritual cleansing—are routinely performed as a symbol of reconciliation when a former LRA member returns home. Such community-level interventions are great platforms for psychosocial healing, building trust, and strengthening solidarity, but the exclusion of women and girls in what is considered a male domain breeds inequity. Even then, women rise up and demonstrate their commitment to community rebuilding. Where there is breakdown of the family unit, they come together and share experiences through storytelling and entertainment as a way to seek and give support to each other. Through government-aided programs, many engage in skills training for self-reliance, and girls attend school. Policy-level interventions that focus on attracting broader stakeholder support in key areas such as psychosocial health, education, employment, and training of community health workers have also been key to improving the quality of life. However, some challenges still persist because of limited resource allocation and the lack of political will. In 2009, the Lango war claimants took the Government of Uganda to court for failing to pay reparations for livestock and property that were looted by the Government Army and the LRA during the prolonged conflict. The defendant retaliated by claiming that funds had been diverted to prioritize development of industrial parks, durable roads, and wealth creation. A decade later, funds were released, but most claimants missed out on compensation because of a deliberately frustrating bureaucratic process.

The people of northern Uganda have embraced the spirit of forgiveness, shown resilience, and moved toward development in the 10 years since peace returned to the region. According to the World Health Organization, the health of all people is fundamental to the attainment of peace and security and is dependent on the fullest co-operation of individuals and states. In this regard, the Government of Uganda, the perpetrators of the LRA conflict, local stakeholders, and victims have made progress toward peace-building for reconciliation and recovery. AJPH

CORRESPONDENCE

Correspondence should be sent to Susan Awor, PO Box 28019, Kampala, Uganda (e-mail: susanawor@berkeley.edu). Reprints can be ordered at http://www.ajph.org by clicking the "Reprints" link.

PUBLICATION INFORMATION

Full Citation: Awor S. Pathways to peace and public health equity among women and children in conflict zones: the case of northern Uganda. *Am J Public Health*. 2023;113(2):158–159.

Acceptance Date: November 18, 2022.

DOI: https://doi.org/10.2105/AJPH.2022.307183

ACKNOWLEDGMENTS

Heartfelt gratitude to Evan vanDommelen Gonzalez for her mentorship and support.

CONFLICTS OF INTEREST

The author declares no conflicts of interest.

REFERENCES

1. Littman RJ. The plague of Athens: epidemiology and paleopathology. *Mt Sinai J Med*. 2009;76(5):456–467. https://doi.org/10.1002/msj.20137
2. Byerly CR. The US military and the influenza pandemic of 1918–1919. *Public Health Rep*. 2010;125(suppl 3):81–91.
3. Buvinic M, Das Gupta M, Casabonne U, Verwimp P. Violent conflict and gender inequality: an overview. *World Bank Res Obs*. 2013;28(1):110–138.
4. UNSCR 1325. In: Richmond OP, Visoka G, eds. *The Palgrave Encyclopedia of Peace and Conflict Studies*. London, UK: Palgrave Macmillan; 2022:1629. https://doi.org/10.1007/978-3-030-77954-2_300695
5. Link BG, Phelan J. Social conditions as fundamental causes of disease. *J Health Soc Behav*. 1995;35(spec no.):80–94.
6. Justice and Reconciliation Project. "The cooling of hearts": community truth-telling in Acholi-Land. Justice and Reconciliation Project. August 4, 2011. Available at: http://www.justiceandreconciliation.org/publications/reports/2007/the-cooling-of-hearts-community-truth-telling-in-acholi-land. Accessed October 27, 2022.

The Visibility of Evictions (an Image of Health)

Eric Persaud, DrPH, MEA

An eviction mortarium was put in place in response to the COVID-19 pandemic that helped reduce New York statewide eviction totals to 3059 in 2020, compared with approximately 17 000 evictions in 2019.[1,2] The eviction mortarium expired on January 16, 2022, and New York City saw a resurgence of evictions being filed.[3]

Such evictions dislodge people from their homes and contribute to the national homelessness crisis, for example, an estimated 326 000 people in 2021 were sheltered. That total includes only people found in shelters, transitional housing, and other temporary housing environments.[4]

At a time when rent and inflation are increasing and labor wages remain stagnant, more and more Americans are being pushed into homelessness by eviction. Legal systems are working to train lawyers and are hiring lawyers to handle surges in eviction cases. However, rather than thus seeking to profit on evictions, the evictions should be prevented in the first place. Families struggling to pay rent brought on by the hardships of the COVID-19 pandemic and economic barriers need legal protection, not punishment. AJPH

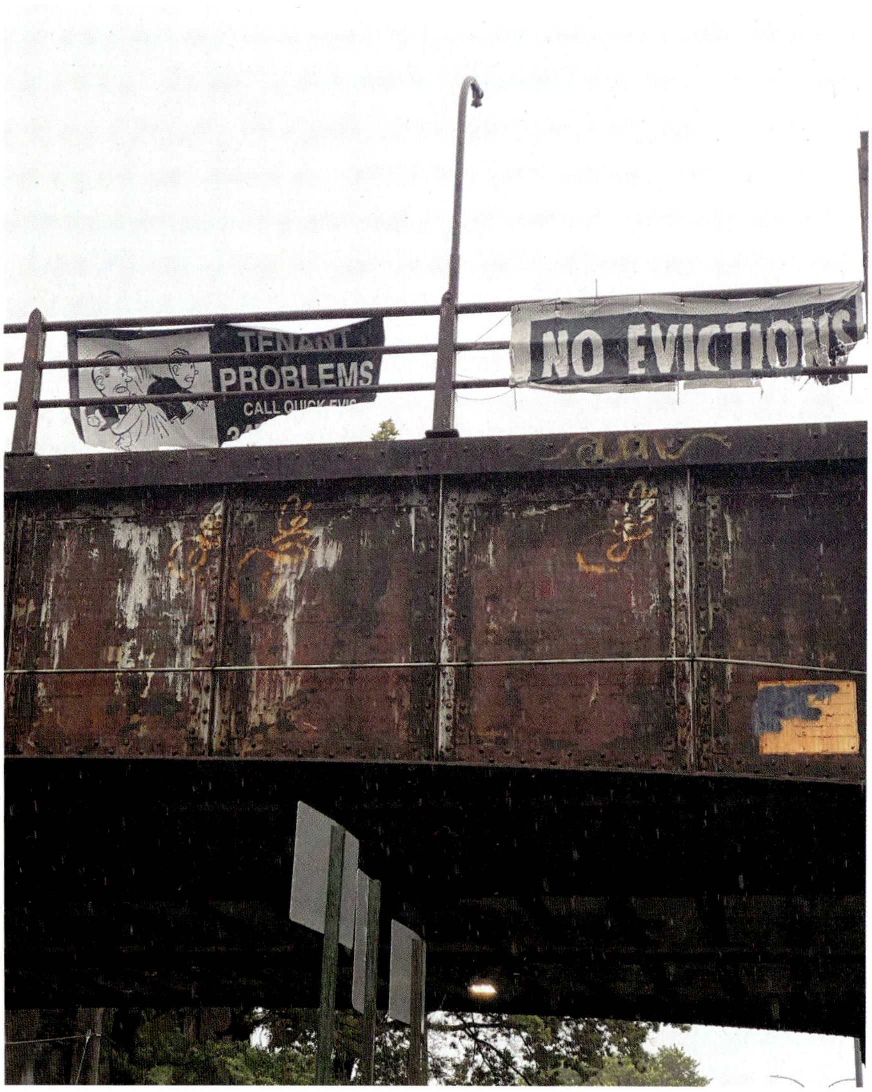

FIGURE 1— Two banners hang side by side along a freeway overpass, fluttering on a rainy day in Queens, New York. To the left is an advertisement that says "tenant problems" with an image of one man kicking the other. There was a telephone number below the text that may have been ripped off. To the right, also in black-and-white, is the other banner, which says, "no evictions," which appears to have been tattered by weather.

ABOUT THE AUTHOR

Eric Persaud is an occupational health researcher and evaluator.

CORRESPONDENCE

Correspondence should be sent to Eric Persaud, 109-03 103rd Ave, South Richmond Hill, NY 11419 (e-mail: epersau01@gmail.com). Reprints can be ordered at http://www.ajph.org by clicking the "Reprints" link.

PUBLICATION INFORMATION

Full Citation: Persaud E. The visibility of evictions (an image of health). *Am J Public Health* 2023;113(2):160–161.

Acceptance Date: November 16, 2022.

DOI: https://doi.org/10.2105/AJPH.2022.307182

ACKNOWLEDGMENTS

I thank the editors for their helpful comments.

CONFLICTS OF INTEREST

The author reports no conflicts of interest.

REFERENCES

1. New York State Governor's Office. Governor Hochul signs new moratorium on COVID-related residential and commercial evictions into law. September 21, 2021. Available at: https://www.governor.ny.gov/news/governor-hochul-signs-new-moratorium-covid-related-residential-and-commercial-evictions-law. Accessed October 2, 2022.
2. Fertig B. NYC evictions dropped by more than 80% in 2020. 2021. Available at: https://beta.gothamist.com/news/nyc-evictions-dropped-more-80-2020?betaRedirect=true. Accessed October 2, 2022.
3. Zaveri M. After a two-year dip, evictions accelerate in New York. *New York Times*. May 2, 2022. Available at: https://www.nytimes.com/2022/05/02/nyregion/new-york-evictions-cases.html. Accessed October 2, 2022.
4. US Department of Housing and Urban Development. HUD releases 2021 annual homeless assessment report, part 1. February 4, 2022. Available at: https://www.hud.gov/press/press_releases_media_advisories/hud_no_22_022. Accessed October 2, 2022.

Treating Hepatitis C in Individuals With Previous Incarceration: The Veterans Health Administration, 2012–2019

Laura Hawks, MD, MPH, Emily A. Wang, MD, MAS, Adeel A. Butt, MD, MS, Stephen Crystal, PhD, MA, D. Keith McInnes, ScD, MS, Vincent Lo Re III, MD, MSCE, Emily J. Cartwright, MD, Lisa B. Puglisi, MD, Lamia Y. K. Haque, MD, MPH, Joseph K. Lim, MD, Amy C. Justice, MD, PhD, and Kathleen A. McGinnis, DrPH, MS

To determine whether the Veterans Health Administration's (VHA) hepatitis C (HCV) treatment campaign reached marginalized populations, we compared HCV care by previous incarceration status with Veterans Aging Cohort Study data. Of those with and those without previous incarceration, respectively, 40% and 21% had detectable HCV, 59% and 65% underwent treatment ($P = .07$); 92% and 94% of those who completed treatment achieved sustained virologic response. The VHA HCV treatment effort was successful and other systems should replicate those efforts. (*Am J Public Health*. 2023;113(2):162–165. https://doi.org/10.2105/AJPH.2022.307152)

AJPH February 2023, Vol 113, No. 2

The Veterans Health Administration (VHA) is the country's largest provider of hepatitis C (HCV) treatment and has identified universal treatment of patients with HCV as a strategic goal. The VHA has recommended broad testing eligibility and reflex confirmation testing since at least 2012.[1] Treatment eligibility has been expanded to include patients regardless of fibrosis stage or comorbid substance use disorders, and treatment is provided at minimal out-of-pocket cost.[1]

INTERVENTION AND IMPLEMENTATION

The VHA developed hepatitis C innovation teams to identify and minimize barriers to treatment of difficult to reach populations by implementing direct outreach programs, increasing staffing for patients experiencing homelessness, expanding pharmacy prescribing privileges, expanding telehealth services, and integrating HCV treatment into opioid treatment programs.[2] As of December 2017, the VHA treated approximately 70% of all those across their system with HCV viremia.[3]

Although engaging difficult to reach populations was a goal of the program, we do not know whether VHA efforts resulted in equitable HCV screening, treatment, and outcomes among disenfranchised populations. Individuals with previous incarceration have disproportionately higher rates of HCV but experience myriad barriers to health care, including decreased access to employment and health insurance, social instability, and discrimination in the health system.[4] Previous incarceration is associated with worse health outcomes in other chronic diseases, including HIV and hypertension,[5,6] thus examining their outcomes would provide a strong indicator of equitable access to care in the VHA.

PLACE, TIME, AND PERSONS

The Veterans Aging Cohort Study (VACS) survey sample is part of an ongoing national observational cohort study of veterans in care with and without HIV at eight sites. Our analytic sample included 1632 participants with and 1477 without HIV who completed a survey between October 2012 and June 2019, answered the survey question about the personal history of incarceration, and were born between 1945 and 1965. Of the 3109 participants in the analytic sample, 96% were male, 64% Black, 27% White, and 8% Hispanic; their ages ranged from 49 to 70 years.

PURPOSE

After the development of a highly effective and tolerated treatment of HCV, the VHA pursued a goal of universal treatment in an effort to eradicate HCV in its patient population.[2] To understand whether individuals with previous incarceration were included in these efforts, we used data from VACS to compare the HCV treatment cascade steps between those with and those without previous incarceration. Because the cohort was initially designed to study HIV, we also ran analyses comparing the treatment cascade steps between those with and those without HIV, stratified by previous incarceration status.

EVALUATION AND ADVERSE EFFECTS

We linked VACS data to the VHA electronic health records, including laboratory and pharmacy data, via the Clinical Data Warehouse; the methods have been described elsewhere.[7] We included these HCV treatment cascade steps[8]: HCV screening, viral load (VL) confirmation, initiation of direct-acting antiviral (DAA) treatment starting January 1, 2014 (the year DAAs became available), completion of DAA treatment by February 19, 2019, VL suppression at last test, and sustained virologic response (SVR). All participants were eligible for screening per the US Preventive Service Task Force recommendations during the study period, using HCV antibody or RNA polymerase chain reaction VL tests.

We considered those with a positive VL to have chronic HCV and to be eligible for DAA treatment. DAA initiation was based on receiving at least one DAA medication fill in the VHA. We identified DAA completion by patients having at least eight weeks of DAA medication filled in the VHA, the minimum recommended time according to guidelines.[9] We measured VL suppression at last test because more than 90% with undetectable VL after treatment completion will remain so at 12 weeks, but some may not return for follow-up lab testing.[10] We considered SVR achieved by the presence of an undetectable VL at least 12 weeks after treatment completion, reflecting current clinical guidelines.

Of the 3109 VACS participants included in this study, 1817 (58%) reported a history of incarceration. HCV screening was conducted in 99% of those with and those without previous incarceration; and VL confirmation occurred for 99% and 98% of those with and those without previous incarceration, respectively. HCV prevalence was 40% and 21% among those with and those without previous incarceration, respectively ($P < .001$). Figure 1 shows the treatment cascade by previous incarceration among the 993 patients eligible for treatment. Among those with HCV, 599 (60%) underwent treatment (59% previous incarceration, 65% without previous incarceration; $P = .07$), and 541 (55%) completed therapy (53% previous incarceration, 59% without previous incarceration; $P = .11$). The treatment cascade was also similar by HIV status (Figure 2).

Of the 599 who initiated treatment, 90% for those with and those without previous incarceration completed eight weeks of treatment. Of the 541 who completed eight weeks of treatment, more than 98% had VL suppression at last test and 93% achieved SVR (92% previous incarceration, 94% without previous incarceration; $P = .58$).

SUSTAINABILITY

This model can serve as an example for other health care systems to achieve high rates of HCV cure. Tactics that can be applied to other systems include broad testing and treatment eligibility and reflex testing for positive screens, expanding prescribing privileges to include pharmacists, broadening telehealth services, integrating HCV treatment into opioid treatment programs and homeless shelters, and minimizing cost sharing.

PUBLIC HEALTH SIGNIFICANCE

Amid a historic effort to reduce barriers to HCV care in the VHA, HCV cascade outcomes were similar among those with and those without self-reported previous incarceration in those born from 1945 to 1965 and participating in VACS. Screening and confirmation of HCV occurred in more than 98% of cases including among those with previous incarceration, which is substantially higher than other published screening rates.[11] DAA initiation, treatment completion, and viral suppression were slightly lower for those with previous incarceration than those without previous incarceration, but the differences were not statistically significant. Of those who initiated treatment, a high and similar percentage (> 90%) in those with and those without previous incarceration completed treatment and achieved SVR. Future research should also evaluate whether the treatment cascade differs by region or recent incarceration.

The VHA's provision of universal and systematized delivery of HCV treatment can be used as a model for increasing both resources and

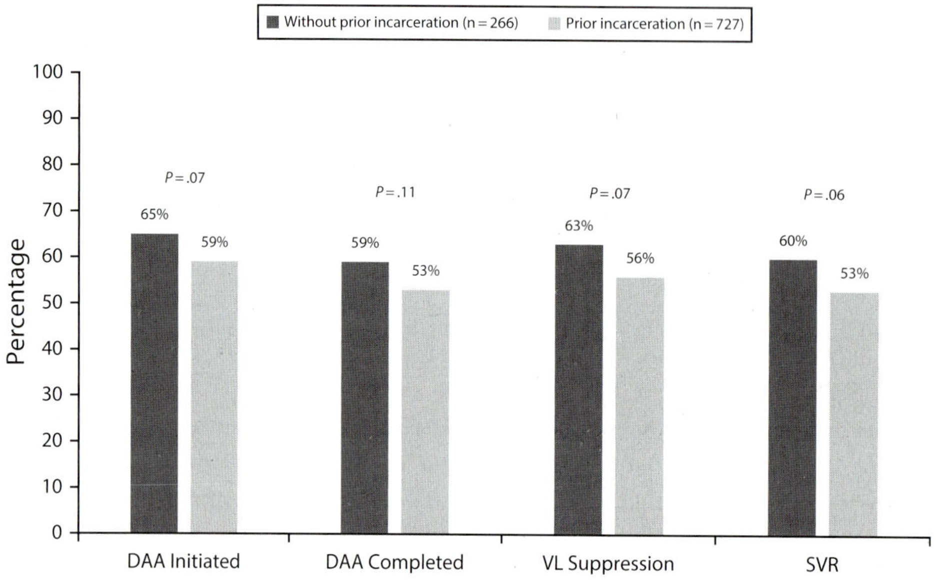

FIGURE 1— HCV Treatment Cascade by Previous Incarceration Status Among Those in the Veterans Aging Cohort Study Survey Sample With Confirmed Chronic HCV: United States, October 2012–June 2019

Note. DAA = direct-acting antiviral; HCV = hepatitis C; SVR = sustained virologic response at 12 wk; VL = viral load. Study population size was n = 993.

public health infrastructure to combat HCV and other infectious diseases, in addition to reducing disparities. For the United States to achieve the World Health Organization's goal of HCV eradication by 2030, urgent attention should be paid to understanding which VHA-initiated efforts could be replicated in other health care systems or used for public health strategies outside the VHA. *AJPH*

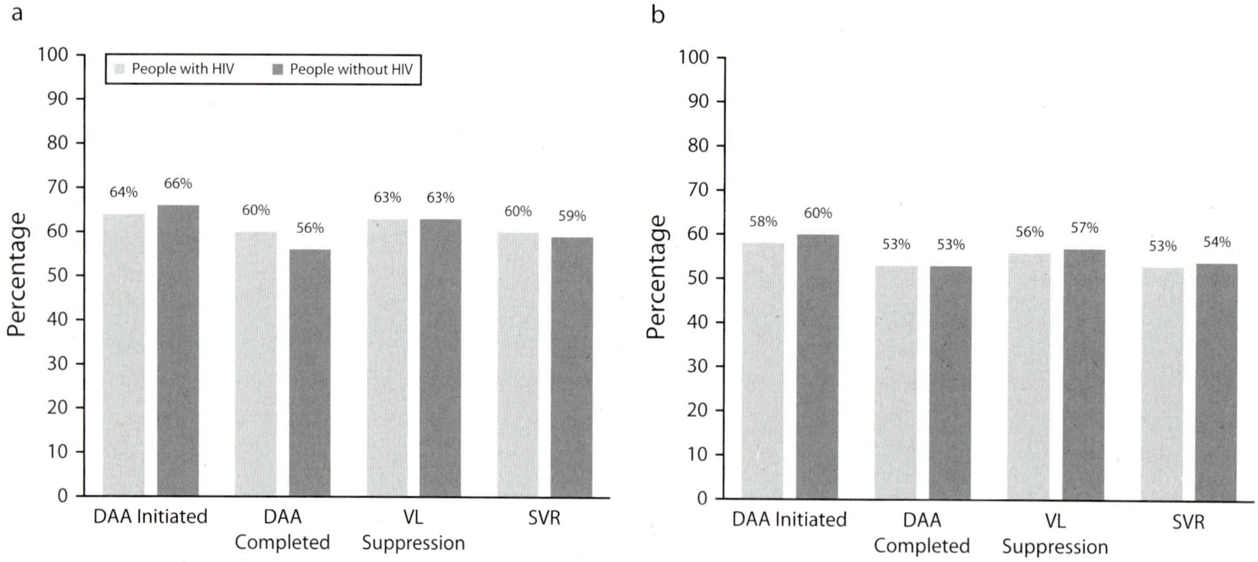

FIGURE 2— HCV Treatment Cascade by HIV Among Those in the Veterans Aging Cohort Study Survey Sample With Confirmed Chronic HCV and (a) Without Prior Incarceration and (b) With Prior Incarceration: United States, October 2012–June 2019

Note. DAA = direct-acting antiviral; HCV = hepatitis C; SVR = sustained virologic response at 12 wk; VL = viral load. Study population size was n = 993. There were no statistically significant differences in the treatment cascade steps by HIV status (all $P \geq .5$).

ABOUT THE AUTHORS

Laura Hawks is with the Center for Advancing Population Science, Medical College of Wisconsin, Milwaukee. Emily A. Wang and Lisa B. Puglisi are with the SEICHE Center for Health and Justice, Yale School of Medicine, New Haven, CT. Adeel A. Butt is with the Department of Medicine, Weill Cornell Medical College, New York, NY. Stephen Crystal is with the Center for Health Services Research, Rutgers University, New Brunswick, NJ. D. Keith McInnes is with the Department of Health Law, Policy, and Management, Boston University School of Public Health, Boston, MA. Vincent Lo Re III is with the Department of Medicine, Perelman School of Medicine, University of Pennsylvania, Philadelphia. Emily J. Cartwright is with the Department of Medicine, Emory University School of Medicine, Atlanta, GA. Lamia Y. K. Haque and Joseph K. Lim are with the Department of Medicine, Yale School of Medicine, New Haven, CT. Amy C. Justice and Kathleen A. McGinnis are with the VA Connecticut Healthcare System, West Haven.

CORRESPONDENCE

Correspondence should be sent to Laura Hawks, MD, MPH, Medical College of Wisconsin, Division of General Internal Medicine, 8701 Watertown Plank Rd, Milwaukee, WI 53226-3596 (e-mail: Lhawks@mcw.edu). Reprints can be ordered at http://www.ajph.org by clicking the "Reprints" link.

PUBLICATION INFORMATION

Full Citation: Hawks L, Wang EA, Butt AA, et al. Treating hepatitis C in individuals with previous incarceration: the veterans health administration, 2012–2019. *Am J Public Health*. 2023;113(2): 162–165.

Acceptance Date: October 10, 2022.

DOI: https://doi.org/10.2105/AJPH.2022.307152

CONTRIBUTORS

L. Hawks drafted and designed the tables and figures and wrote the first draft of the article. L. Hawks, E. A. Wang, A. C. Justice, and K. A. McGinnis conceptualized the study design. L. Hawks and K. A. McGinnis verified the underlying data. K. McInnes analyzed the data. All authors approved the final study design, contributed to reviewing and editing the final draft, had access to the data, and accept responsibility to submit the article for publication.

ACKNOWLEDGMENTS

The study was funded in part by the National Institute on Alcohol Abuse and Alcoholism (grants U24 AA020794, U01 AA020790, U10 AA013566). The study data were presented at the Society of General Internal Medicine National Meeting, April 2021.

CONFLICTS OF INTEREST

The authors have no conflicts of interest or financial disclosures.

HUMAN PARTICIPANT PROTECTION

The institutional review boards at all eight VACS locations (Atlanta, GA; Baltimore, MD; Bronx, NY; New York City, NY; Houston, TX; Los Angeles, CA; Pittsburgh, PA; and Washington, DC) approved this study. All participants provided written consent before enrollment.

REFERENCES

1. Belperio PS, Chartier M, Ross DB, Alaigh P, Shulkin D. Curing hepatitis C virus infection: best practices from the US Department of Veterans Affairs. *Ann Intern Med*. 2017;167(7):499–504. https://doi.org/10.7326/M17-1073
2. Gonzalez R, Park A, Yakovchenko V, et al. HCV elimination in the US Department of Veterans Affairs. *Clin Liver Dis (Hoboken)*. 2021;18(1):1–6. https://doi.org/10.1002/cld.1150
3. Belperio PS, Chartier M, Gonzalez RI, et al. Hepatitis C care in the Department of Veterans Affairs: building a foundation for success. *Infect Dis Clin North Am*. 2018;32(2):281–292. https://doi.org/10.1016/j.idc.2018.02.011
4. Nowotny KM, Kuptsevych-Timmer A. Health and justice: framing incarceration as a social determinant of health for Black men in the United States. *Sociology Compass*. 2018;12(3): e12566. https://doi.org/10.1111/soc4.12566
5. Howell BA, Long JB, Edelman EJ, et al. Incarceration history and uncontrolled blood pressure in a multi-site cohort. *J Gen Intern Med*. 2016;31(12): 1496–1502. https://doi.org/10.1007/s11606-016-3857-1
6. Iroh PA, Mayo H, Nijhawan AE. The HIV care cascade before, during, and after incarceration: a systematic review and data synthesis. *Am J Public Health*. 2015;105(7):e5–e16. https://doi.org/10.2105/AJPH.2015.302635. [Erratum in: *Am J Public Health*. 2018;108(3):e18].
7. Justice AC, Dombrowski E, Conigliaro J, et al. Veterans Aging Cohort Study (VACS): overview and description. *Med Care*. 2006;44(8 suppl 2):S13–S24. https://doi.org/10.1097/01.mlr.0000223741.02074.66
8. Maier MM, Ross DB, Chartier M, Belperio PS, Backus LI. Cascade of care for hepatitis C virus infection within the US Veterans Health Administration. *Am J Public Health*. 2016;106(2):353–358. https://doi.org/10.2105/AJPH.2015.302927
9. American Association for the Study of Liver Diseases; Infectious Diseases Society of America. Simplified HCV Treatment Algorithm for Treatment-Naive Adults Without Cirrhosis. 2020. Available at: https://www.hcvguidelines.org/treatment-naive/simplified-treatment. Accessed March 31, 2021.
10. Corcorran MA, Kim HN. Monitoring during and after HCV treatment. October 12, 2020. Available at: https://www.hepatitisc.uw.edu/go/treatment-infection/monitoring/core-concept/all. Accessed March 31, 2021.
11. Rodriguez CV, Rubenstein KB, Linas B, Hu H, Horberg M. Increasing hepatitis C screening in a large integrated health system: science and policy in concert. *Am J Manag Care*. 2018;24(5): e134–e140.

CDC-Supported National Network of Farmworker-Serving Organizations to Mitigate COVID-19

Bethany Boggess, PhD, Sarah Prager, MPH, Jennifer M. Lincoln, PhD, CSP, Ninel Espinosa Foss, Lic., Edward Kissam, BA, Sylvia Partida, MA, and Alfonso Rodriguez Lainz, PhD, DVM, MPVM

The Centers for Disease Control and Prevention has partnered with the National Center for Farmworker Health to respond to the impact of COVID-19 on US farmworker communities. Immigrant farmworkers are often isolated from public health infrastructure. This partnership built the capacity of a national network of organizations to connect farmworkers to COVID-19 education and vaccinations in 20 states through training and resource sharing. The partnership funded 194 network member staff, trained 1130 individuals, and supported COVID-19 outreach to more than 600 000 farmworkers. (*Am J Public Health*. 2023;113(2):166–169. https://doi.org/10.2105/AJPH.2022.307159)

AJPH February 2023, Vol 113, No. 2

Farmworkers were considered to be essential during the COVID-19 pandemic, but they experienced numerous inequities throughout the different pandemic phases.[1–5] The 2.5 million US farmworkers are primarily immigrants, with more than two thirds born outside of the United States and half lacking authorization to work in the country.[6,7] Farmworkers have been found to have a four times higher incidence of COVID-19 infection than nonfarmworkers.[4] Such health disparities are associated with vulnerabilities including crowded housing, lack of paid time off, limited access to health care, ineligibility for most federal public benefits, and an elevated prevalence of certain health risk factors for severe COVID-19 symptoms (e.g., diabetes).[8–10]

The ill-equipped public health infrastructure in the rural United States exacerbated existing disparities during the pandemic.[11] Many community-based organizations around the country quickly stepped up to meet the needs of farmworkers, but they often had limited capacity and resources to address needs. The purpose of this article is to describe the initial impact of the development of a national network focused on protecting farmworkers' health during the pandemic.

INTERVENTION AND IMPLEMENTATION

To help address public health infrastructure gaps among farmworkers, the Centers for Disease Control and Prevention (CDC) established a partnership with and provided $7.8 million in funding to the National Center for Farmworker Health (NCFH). NCFH established a national network of farmworker-serving organizations to guide and implement the project. The partnership provided COVID-19 prevention guidance to farmworker families and emphasized building the capacity of farmworker-serving organizations to conduct COVID-19-related outreach and education and support vaccination distribution.

Project implementation was guided by an advisory council that included farmworkers, employers, researchers, and organizational representatives. Twenty members were selected on the basis of multiple factors to ensure diversity in geography, areas of expertise, and organizational missions. Ten of the members were also funded network subrecipients. The council provided monthly guidance on project priorities. CDC staff provided technical support and facilitated coordination with the CDC COVID-19 response.

The primary strategy was to enhance the organizational capacity of the network partners through training, resources, and funding. The subcontract language was flexible so that organizations could implement local strategies using their own expertise. On the basis of needs identified from capacity assessments, NCFH provided responsive training and technical

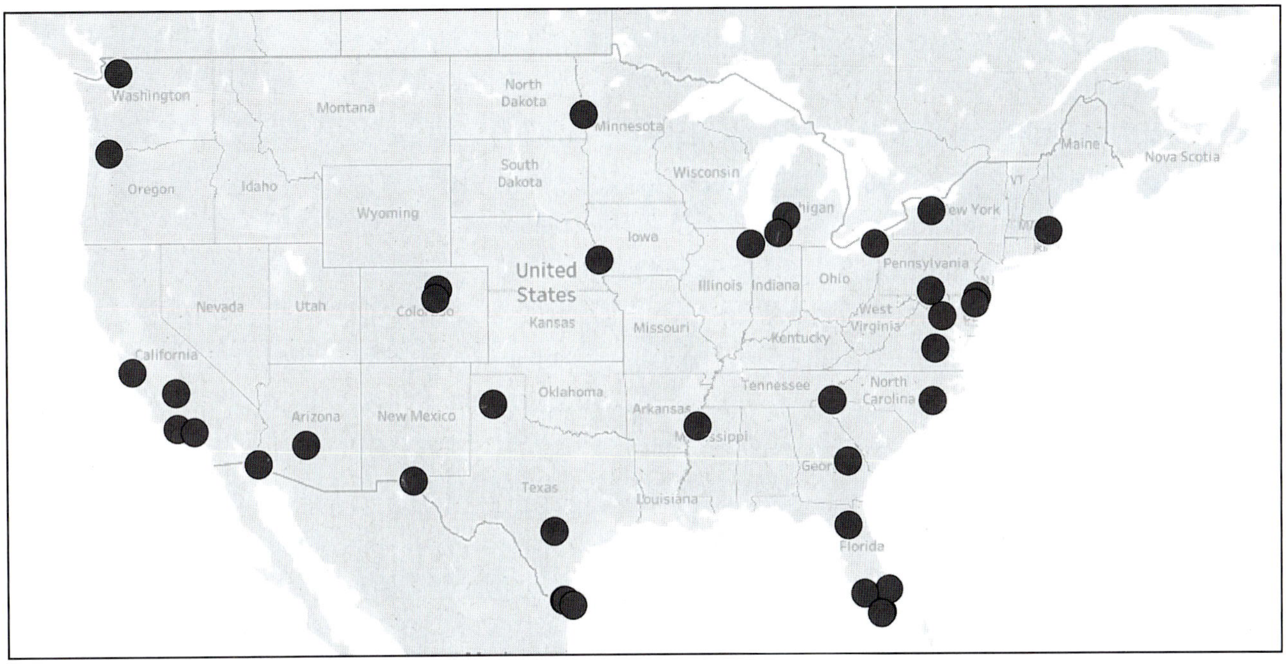

FIGURE 1— **Location of 41 Farmworker-Serving Network Organizations That Received Technical Assistance as Part of the CDC/NCFH Partnership to Protect and Support Farmworkers During the COVID-19 Pandemic, October 2020–September 2021**

Note. CDC = Centers for Disease Control and Prevention; NCFH = National Center for Farmworker Health.

assistance (TA) sessions, disseminated resources, and supported the development of new partnerships.

PLACE, TIME, AND PERSONS

The project, which was national in scope and implemented from October 2020 through September 2021, focused on geographic areas with high concentrations of farmworkers. Network partners were located in 20 states (Figure 1).

There were 54 network partners formally involved in the project. Forty-one organizations were formally subcontracted to provide COVID-19 outreach, education, mitigation, and vaccination support. Two of the organizations were agricultural employers, and the remaining 39 were providers of social, health, or legal services to farmworkers.

PURPOSE

The partnership was established with the following objectives: (1) enhance the capacity of farmworker-serving organizations to connect farmworkers and their families to COVID-19 education, resources, and vaccines and (2) build a network to increase collaboration among farmworker-serving organizations and other entities as a means of enhancing the impact and sustainability of their efforts.

EVALUATION AND ADVERSE EFFECTS

To assess the initial impact of the project, network organizations regularly reported quantitative data on their activities to NCFH. NCFH collected data via capacity assessments, virtual meetings, telephone interviews, and surveys regarding needs and experiences during the project.

Advisory Council

Ninety percent of members felt that their voice was always heard during meetings and acted on by NCFH. Council member input was often actionable; for example, members recommended supporting local vaccination efforts over national campaigns, and when NCFH received additional funds for the project, support for local vaccination efforts was prioritized.

Capacity Assessment and Training

Key needs identified in organizational capacity assessments included themes such as outreach with vaccine-hesitant farmworkers, social media usage, and virus variants, among others. NCFH directly connected organizations that needed expertise in a certain area with organizations that possessed such expertise.

In response to broadly identified information or capacity needs, NCFH hosted 11 virtual English- and Spanish-language training sessions for 1130 participants from farmworker-serving organizations. The overall objective of the training was to increase outreach and public health knowledge while building on participants' existing knowledge of their local communities. Training evaluations indicated increases in knowledge: 65% of the participants reported a high or extremely high level of knowledge gained, and 89% were satisfied or extremely satisfied with the training they received.

TABLE 1— Summary of Project Outcomes Resulting From the CDC/NCFH Network Partnership to Protect and Support Farmworkers During the COVID-19 Pandemic, October 2020–September 2021

Outcome[a]	No.
Capacity-building activities	
Full- or part-time staff supported through network funds	194
Network training participants	1 130
Technical assistance support recipients	1 107
Farmworker outreach activities	
Farmworkers and family members who received at least one dose of a COVID-19 vaccine	63 290
Farmworkers and family members reached with COVID-19 prevention or vaccine education (in person, via telephone, or through video calls)[b]	601 956
Facemasks, gloves, hand sanitizer items distributed to farmworkers	568 320
Farmworkers who received COVID-19 testing referrals and support	46 389
Farmworkers who received food distribution or isolation and quarantine support	10 016

Note. CDC = Centers for Disease Control and Prevention; NCFH = National Center for Farmworker Health.

[a]Some individuals may have received more than one service. Because of differences in the timeline to complete subcontracts, six organizations reported metrics from November 2020 through September 2021 and 35 organizations reported metrics from May 2021 through September 2021. The metrics reported here reflect all metrics reported from November 2020 through September 2021.

[b]Two organizations were able to report only all farmworkers educated by their organization and not the number reached specifically through activities undertaken pursuant to the CDC/NCFH cooperative agreement and the NCFH subcontracts.

Staff and Outreach Resources

Project funds supported 194 part-time and full-time outreach and programmatic staff. Organizations reported reaching 601 956 farmworkers and family members with COVID-19 education through telephonic, video, or face-to-face methods (some individuals may have received more than one service) and assisted in providing at least one dose of a COVID-19 vaccine to more than 63 290 farmworkers and family members during the project period. Organizations also were given multilingual health education materials and face masks, gloves, and hand sanitizer to distribute to farmworkers (Table 1).

Technical Assistance

In addition to group training, NCFH provided TA support to organizations to build their capacity and increase access to public health resources. Types of TA included identifying health education resources appropriate for farmworkers, presenting at workshops, exchanging ideas among partners, and offering support in using outreach technologies. A total of 1017 individuals took part in nearly 230 TA interactions focused on COVID-19.

Network Collaborations

Supporting collaborations among farmworker-serving organizations, employers and industry associations, health departments, and CDC programs was another major focus of building capacity. Connecting new partners was facilitated via local network projects, TA interactions, and hosting of network calls to exchange ideas, build skills, and learn about promising practices around the country. NCFH hosted a total of eight network calls in English and Spanish, and an average of 22 participants attended each call. This exchange of ideas was especially critical for innovation and problem solving when organizations were dealing with widespread outbreaks of COVID-19 and during earlier phases of vaccine distribution.

SUSTAINABILITY

Network members indicated that partnership resources were essential to provide COVID-19 education to farmworkers and support vaccination efforts. The primary challenges in implementing these efforts were rapidly evolving public health strategies and limited capacity of local organizations as a result of other projects or staff shortages. Sustaining the staffing levels and resources used to maintain the network is projected to cost $4 million to reach approximately 600 000 farmworkers and their families annually. Continuing the network would facilitate ongoing outreach and education on a variety of health topics and a more rapid response to future public health emergencies.

PUBLIC HEALTH SIGNIFICANCE

We concluded that local farmworker-serving organizations played a critical role in implementing public health activities during the pandemic through disseminating public health information and guidance, bringing local issues among farmworkers to the attention of public health officials, and delivering health services and education to farmworkers. A national partnership focused on allowing local organizations to act on their expertise may be useful in efforts to address other health needs of farmworkers and reduce health disparities faced by this critically important population. AJPH

ABOUT THE AUTHORS

Bethany Boggess, Sarah Prager, and Sylvia Partida are with the National Center for Farmworker Health, Buda, TX. Jennifer M. Lincoln and Alfonso Rodriguez Lainz are with the Centers for Disease Control and Prevention, Atlanta, GA. Ninel Espinosa Foss is with the Central Virginia Legal Aid Society, Richmond, VA. Edward Kissam is with the Werner-Kohnstamm Family Giving Fund, Oakland, CA.

CORRESPONDENCE

Correspondence should be sent to Bethany Boggess, PhD, 1770 FM 967, Buda, TX 78610 (e-mail: bcboggess@gmail.com). Reprints can be ordered at http://www.ajph.org by clicking the "Reprints" link.

PUBLICATION INFORMATION

Full Citation: Boggess B, Prager S, Lincoln JM, et al. CDC-supported national network of farmworker-serving organizations to mitigate COVID-19. *Am J Public Health*. 2023;113(2):166–169.

Acceptance Date: October 17, 2022.

DOI: https://doi.org/10.2105/AJPH.2022.307159

CONTRIBUTORS

B. Boggess contributed to the design of the network evaluation, evaluation conceptualization, and data analysis and drafted the original content. S. Prager contributed to the design of the network evaluation, evaluation conceptualization, and data analysis and provided feedback on original content. J. M. Lincoln, N. E. Foss, and E. Kissam reviewed and provided critical revisions to content. S. Partida and A. R. Lainz contributed to the design of the network evaluation and provided critical feedback to content.

ACKNOWLEDGMENTS

This program was funded by the Centers for Disease Control and Prevention (cooperative agreement CK-20-2003).

We are deeply grateful to the farmworkers who have continued to provide food throughout the pandemic and to the organizations that have worked tirelessly to serve and advocate for them. We are grateful to Emma Torres of Campesinos Sin Fronteras, Genevieve Flores-Haro of the Mixteco/Indigena Community Organizing Project, Irene de Barraicua of Lideres Campesinas, and Matt Solberg of the National Center for Farmworker Health for their support on this article. We also acknowledge the work of Katharina C. Whitsett, Yvette Salinas, Erin Birney, Lisbeth Gall, and Elvia Anderson, who supported network organizations and led evaluation data collection efforts.

Note. The findings and conclusions in this report are those of the authors and do not necessarily represent the official position of the Centers for Disease Control and Prevention.

CONFLICTS OF INTEREST

The authors have no conflicts of interest to disclose.

HUMAN PARTICIPANT PROTECTION

Institutional review board approval was not required because this study did not include any human participant research data.

REFERENCES

1. Kissam E. The impact of the COVID-19 pandemic on California farmworkers: better local data collection and reporting will improve strategic response. *Stat J IAOS*. 2020;36(4):867–898. https://doi.org/10.3233/SJI-200763
2. Lusk JL, Chandra R. Farmer and farm worker illnesses and deaths from COVID-19 and impacts on agricultural output. *PLoS One*. 2021;16(4):e0250621. https://doi.org/10.1371/journal.pone.0250621
3. Riley AR, Chen YH, Matthay EC, et al. Excess mortality among Latino people in California during the COVID-19 pandemic. *SSM Popul Health*. 2021;15:100860. https://doi.org/10.1016/j.ssmph.2021.100860
4. Mora AM, Lewnard JA, Kogut K, et al. Risk factors associated with SARS-CoV-2 infection among farmworkers in Monterey County, California. *JAMA Netw Open*. 2021;4(9):e2124116. https://doi.org/10.1001/jamanetworkopen.2021.24116
5. Ramirez S, Mines R, Carlisle-Cummins I. COVID-19 Farmworker Study. Available at: https://cirsinc.org/covid-19-farmworker-study. Accessed January 5, 2022.
6. US Department of Agriculture, Economic Research Service. Farm labor. Available at: https://www.ers.usda.gov/topics/farm-economy/farm-labor/#size. Accessed January 5, 2022.
7. Ornelas I, Fung W, Gabbard S, Carroll D. Findings from the National Agricultural Workers Survey (NAWS) 2017–2018: a demographic and employment profile of United States farmworkers. Available at: https://wdr.doleta.gov/research/FullText_Documents/ETAOP2021-22%20NAWS%20Research%20Report%2014%20(2017-2018)_508%20Compliant.pdf. Accessed January 5, 2022.
8. Ramos AK. A human rights-based approach to farmworker health: an overarching framework to address the social determinants of health. *J Agromedicine*. 2018;23(1):25–31. https://doi.org/10.1080/1059924X.2017.1384419
9. O'Halloran AC, Lu PJ, Williams WW, et al. Influenza vaccination among workers—21 U.S. states, 2013. *Am J Infect Control*. 2017;45(4):410–416. https://doi.org/10.1016/j.ajic.2017.01.005
10. Moore KL, Mercado J, Hill J, Katz SC. Disparities in health insurance coverage and health status among farmworkers, Sonoma County, California, 2013–2014. *Prev Chronic Dis*. 2016;13:E45. https://doi.org/10.5888/pcd13.150519
11. Raghuveer TS, Kriesel D. Urgent and massive investment in US public health infrastructure will help to stop the spread of SARS-CoV-2 virus and deaths from COVID-19. *Kans J Med*. 2021;14:84–86. https://doi.org/10.17161/kjm.vol1415061

A COVID-19 Vaccination Program to Promote Uptake and Equity for People Experiencing Homelessness in Los Angeles County

Allison D. Rosen, PhD, Alexander Senturia, BA, Isabelle Howerton, MPH, Emily Uyeda Kantrim, BA, Vanessa Evans, MSN, RN, Tiffany Malluche, MSN, RN, Jonni Miller, MSW, Miriam Gonzalez, BA, Brooke Robie, BS, Chelsea L. Shover, PhD, Alicia H. Chang, MD, MS, Heidi Behforouz, MD, Anh Nguyen, MD, MBA, and Emily H. Thomas, MD, MS

People experiencing homelessness (PEH) have been disproportionately affected by COVID-19, yet their vaccination coverage is lower than is that of the general population. We implemented a COVID-19 vaccination program that used evidence-based and culturally tailored approaches to promote vaccine uptake and equity for PEH in Los Angeles County, California. From February 2021 through February 2022, 33 977 doses of vaccine were administered at 2658 clinics, and 9275 PEH were fully vaccinated. This program may serve as a model for future service delivery in vulnerable populations. (*Am J Public Health*. 2023;113(2):170–174. https://doi.org/10.2105/AJPH.2022.307147)

AJPH February 2023, Vol 113, No. 2

To promote COVID-19 vaccination among people experiencing homelessness (PEH), Housing for Health (HFH), a division of the Los Angeles (LA) County Department of Health Services in California, implemented a mobile vaccination program in partnership with the LA County Department of Public Health.

INTERVENTION AND IMPLEMENTATION

We held clinics at shelters, homeless services centers, encampments, and other public spaces. Teams also canvassed areas by car and on foot to identify locations where unsheltered PEH were residing. We visited locations every two to four weeks to provide first, second, and booster doses until saturation of vaccine interest was reached. We offered vaccines from all three pharmaceutical companies that manufacture COVID-19 vaccinations, Moderna, Pfizer, and Janssen, at most clinics.

Teams of nurses, emergency medical technicians, community health workers, and homeless services staff trained in motivational interviewing and trauma-informed care provided vaccine education and administration. Outreach efforts informed by the concept of self-determination and the "whatever it takes" model provided PEH with education and resources to make informed decisions about their health.[1,2] Teams provided food, hygiene kits, tents, and harm reduction supplies to PEH regardless of their interest in vaccination. Community health workers engaged PEH in face-to-face conversations and were trained to invite current PEH, called peer ambassadors, to share personal stories about being vaccinated.[3] Paired with these extensive education efforts, $50 gift cards for first doses and $25 gift cards for subsequent doses were offered to those vaccinated beginning in September 2021.

Teams regularly reviewed data to identify groups that had disparities in uptake, and we used quality improvement studies in the form of rapid field surveys to evaluate outreach strategies and understand reasons for vaccine hesitancy. We then designed educational pamphlets and games to address the most cited reasons for hesitancy.

PLACE, TIME, AND PERSONS

Implementation occurred between February 3, 2021 and February 5, 2022 in LA County. The program primarily served PEH as well as homeless services staff and individuals with housing insecurity or previous homelessness.

PURPOSE

Given the elevated risk of COVID-19 mortality among PEH, access to vaccination is vital for this population.[4] There is a need for programs to bring vaccines directly to shelters and encampments and address the high rates of mistrust of, concern about, and hesitancy toward vaccination among PEH.[5,6] Our program aimed to use evidence-based and culturally tailored approaches to promote COVID-19 vaccine uptake and equity among PEH in LA County.[1,2,6,7]

EVALUATION AND ADVERSE EFFECTS

HFH held 2658 clinics, averaging 51 per week. Of these clinics, 1032 (38.8%) served sheltered PEH and 1626 (61.2%) served unsheltered PEH.

Quality improvement data that we collected beginning in November 2021 revealed that HFH teams engaged more than 1000 PEH in vaccine education weekly; approximately 50% of those engaged participated in quality improvement surveys to evaluate outreach methods. Results suggested that financial incentives were an acceptable strategy: 56% of participants said that being offered a $50 gift card was a primary reason they were vaccinated, whereas 1.7% said they did not get vaccinated because they found it coercive. In addition, 16% of participants cited their conversation with HFH staff as a primary reason for deciding to be vaccinated, highlighting the importance of personal engagement.[8]

HFH administered 33 977 doses of COVID-19 vaccine. PEH received 20 043 (59.0%) doses, homeless services staff received 6199 (18.2%) doses, and individuals with housing insecurity or previous homelessness received 7735 (22.8%) doses. Most doses (n = 17 537; 51.6%) were first doses; 9199 (27.0%) were second doses, 215 (0.6%) were additional doses for immunocompromised individuals, and 7026 (20.7%) were booster doses. The median number of doses per week administered to PEH was 344 (interquartile range = 260–490; Figure 1).

HFH fully vaccinated 9275 PEH; 3564 (38.4%) were sheltered and 5711 (61.6%) were unsheltered. Those fully vaccinated by HFH represent 14.6% (95% confidence interval = 14.3%, 14.8%) of the total unhoused population of LA County (Table 1). In addition, 2052 homeless services staff were fully vaccinated through HFH's program (Table A, available as a supplement to the online version of this article at http://www.ajph.org).

Overall, 4074 (43.9%) of the PEH fully vaccinated by HFH received a two-dose mRNA vaccine, and 66.2% of them returned to an HFH clinic for their

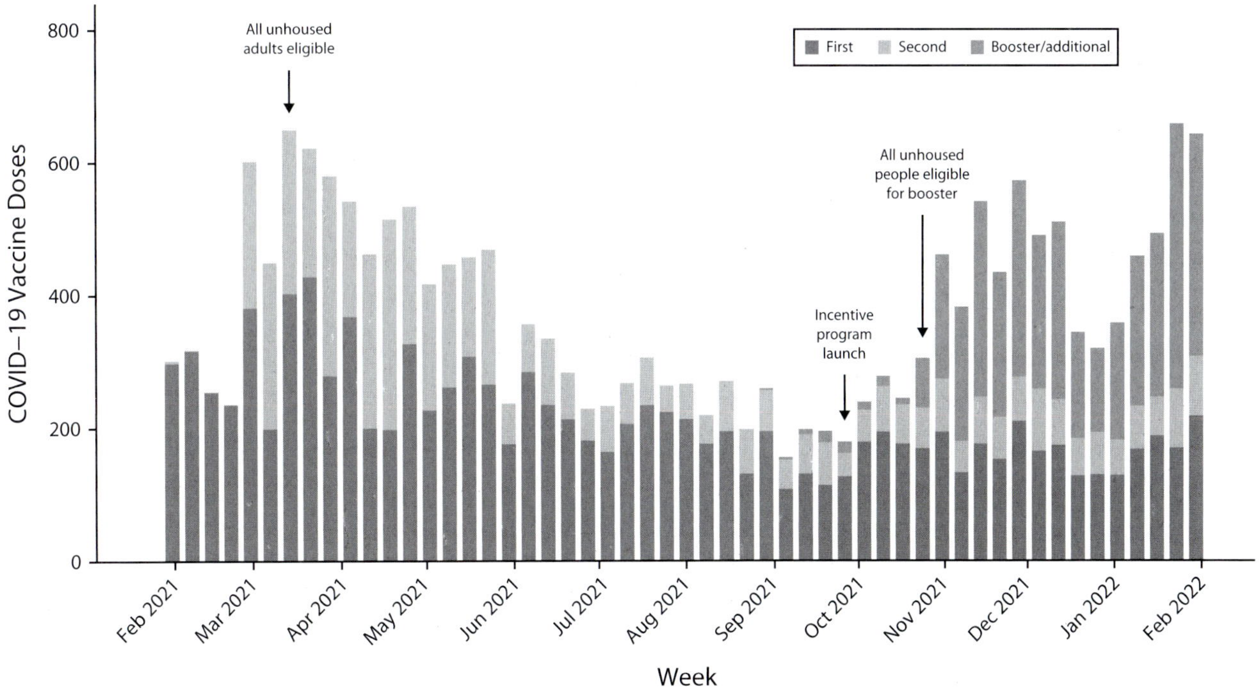

FIGURE 1— Weekly Number of COVID-19 Vaccines Administered to People Experiencing Homelessness by Housing for Health: Los Angeles County, CA, February 3, 2021–February 5, 2022

TABLE 1— People Experiencing Homelessness Fully Vaccinated by Housing for Health: Los Angeles County, CA, February 3, 2021–February 5, 2022

	Total		Sheltered		Unsheltered	
	Vaccinated, No. (%)	Population Size[a] (% Vaccinated)	Vaccinated, No. (%)	Population Size[a] (% Vaccinated)	Vaccinated, No. (%)	Population Size[a] (% Vaccinated)
Total	9275 (100)	63 706 (14.6)	3 564 (100)	17 616 (20.2)	5 711 (100)	46 090 (12.4)
Age, y						
0–17	120 (1.3)	7 491 (1.6)	104 (2.9)	5 863 (1.8)	16 (0.3)	1 628 (1.0)
18–24	330 (3.6)	4 181 (7.9)	155 (4.3)	1 772 (8.7)	175 (3.1)	2 409 (7.3)
25–54	5 094 (54.9)	37 138 (13.7)	1 733 (48.6)	7 135 (24.3)	3 361 (58.9)	30 003 (11.2)
55–61	1 702 (18.4)	8 606 (19.8)	627 (17.6)	1 495 (41.9)	1 075 (18.8)	7 111 (15.1)
≥ 62	2 029 (21.9)	6 290 (32.3)	945 (26.5)	1 351 (69.9)	1 084 (19.0)	4 939 (21.9)
Gender identity[b]						
Male	6 188 (68.2)	42 797 (14.5)	2 200 (63.8)	9 113 (24.1)	3 988 (70.8)	33 684 (11.8)
Female	2 841 (31.3)	20 671 (13.7)	1 239 (35.9)	8 455 (14.7)	1 602 (28.5)	12 216 (13.1)
Nonbinary	9 (0.1)	238 (3.8)	2 (0.1)	48 (4.2)	7 (0.1)	190 (3.7)
Transgender	40 (0.4)	842 (4.8)	7 (0.2)	158 (4.4)	33 (0.6)	684 (4.8)
Race/Ethnicity[c]						
Hispanic/Latino	3 744 (41.7)	23 005 (16.3)	1 299 (37.8)	6 279 (20.7)	2 445 (44.2)	16 726 (14.6)
Non-Hispanic American Indian/Alaska Native	167 (1.9)	686 (24.3)	45 (1.3)	58 (77.6)	122 (2.2)	628 (19.4)
Non-Hispanic Asian	202 (2.3)	774 (26.1)	110 (3.2)	167 (65.9)	92 (1.7)	607 (15.2)
Non-Hispanic Black/ African American	2 537 (28.3)	21 509 (11.8)	1 014 (29.5)	8 424 (12.0)	1 523 (27.5)	13 085 (11.6)
Non-Hispanic Native Hawaiian/ other Pacific Islander	63 (0.7)	205 (30.7)	21 (0.6)	73 (28.8)	42 (0.8)	132 (31.8)
Non-Hispanic other	339 (3.8)	1 319 (25.7)	171 (5.0)	326 (52.5)	168 (3.0)	993 (16.9)
Non-Hispanic White	1 925 (21.4)	16 208 (11.9)	780 (22.7)	2 289 (34.1)	1 145 (20.7)	13 919 (8.2)

[a]We sourced these data from the Los Angeles Homeless Services Authority.[9]
[b]Gender identity was missing for 197 individuals (116 sheltered, 81 unsheltered).
[c]Race/ethnicity was missing for 298 individuals (124 sheltered, 174 unsheltered).

second dose. Among sheltered and unsheltered PEH, second dose follow-up was 79.3% and 53.6%, respectively (Figure A, available as a supplement to the online version of this article at http://www.ajph.org).

To our knowledge, this program did not have any unintended consequences. We reported adverse events to the Vaccine Adverse Events Reporting System; we observed no major adverse events. However, implementation was more challenging among unsheltered PEH, who make up 70% of LA's homeless population.[9] Frequent encampment sweeps fostered government mistrust and made second dose delivery challenging. Additionally, unsheltered PEH reported higher rates of vaccine hesitancy in our quality improvement studies and were twice as likely to be unwilling to engage in education than were sheltered PEH.[8]

SUSTAINABILITY

Mass vaccination campaigns with "hardest to reach" populations are resource intensive. Continued efforts should invest in community-based programs and consider lessons learned from this program. First, health services brought directly to PEH build trust and lasting relationships. Second, programs should invest in staff with lived experience and build stakeholder engagement across elected offices and advocacy groups to facilitate buy-in and drive culturally competent programs. Lastly, responding to a dynamic situation like a pandemic requires real-time data tracking and quality improvement efforts to inform decision-making and resource allocation.

PUBLIC HEALTH SIGNIFICANCE

Amid the rapidly evolving COVID-19 pandemic, HFH designed and implemented a novel program that aimed to increase vaccine uptake and promote equity for PEH. The 9275 PEH fully vaccinated by HFH represent 23.2% of all PEH fully vaccinated in LA County in the year following vaccine rollout.[10]

Uptake and second dose follow-up were consistently higher in sheltered than in unsheltered PEH, although we held 50% more clinics for unsheltered clients. This is likely explained in part by perceived increased COVID-19 risk in congregate settings and by frequent street cleanups that displaced unsheltered PEH.[11]

The program was particularly successful at reaching PEH aged 62 years and older and those who identify as Hispanic/Latino. PEH older than 62 years accounted for 21.9% of HFH vaccinations but represent 9.9% of the homeless population in LA County, and PEH who identify as Hispanic/Latino accounted for 41.7% of HFH vaccinations but represent 36.1% of the population. Continued efforts are needed; the disparities in vaccination observed among PEH vaccinated by HFH mirror those in the entire unhoused and general populations of LA County, suggesting a need for improved strategies to promote vaccination across all populations.[12]

In evaluating our program, we acknowledge that some PEH may have been vaccinated in other settings had this program not existed. However, HFH's low-barrier approach targeted PEH who otherwise would have faced many barriers to vaccination. Anecdotally, we routinely had conversations with individuals who indicated that they would not have otherwise been vaccinated or faced too many barriers in other settings to access vaccination.

Data analyses were limited by the fact that the unhoused population was last counted in early 2020—before the COVID-19 pandemic. Because homelessness likely increased during the pandemic, we may have overestimated the proportion of PEH vaccinated.[9] We likely underestimated the proportion who returned for their second dose of mRNA vaccines, as some may have gotten second doses outside the HFH program.

Much work remains to be done in reducing the burden of COVID-19 among PEH. HFH's innovative program can serve as a model for the ongoing promotion of vaccine uptake and equity in vulnerable populations. AJPH

ABOUT THE AUTHORS

Allison D. Rosen, Alexander Senturia, Isabelle Howerton, Emily Uyeda Kantrim, Vanessa Evans, Tiffany Malluche, Jonni Miller, Miriam Gonzalez, Brooke Robie, Heidi Behforouz, Anh Nguyen, and Emily H. Thomas are with the Los Angeles County Department of Health Services, Los Angeles, CA. Chelsea L. Shover is with the David Geffen School of Medicine, University of California Los Angeles. Alicia H. Chang is with the Los Angeles County Department of Public Health, Los Angeles, CA.

CORRESPONDENCE

Correspondence should be sent to Allison D. Rosen, 10880 Wilshire Blvd, Suite 1800, Los Angeles, CA, 90024 (e-mail: a.rosen@ucla.edu). Reprints can be ordered at http://www.ajph.org by clicking the "Reprints" link.

PUBLICATION INFORMATION

Full Citation: Rosen AD, Senturia A, Howerton I, et al. A COVID-19 vaccination program to promote uptake and equity for people experiencing homelessness in Los Angeles County. *Am J Public Health*. 2023;113(2):170–174.

Acceptance Date: October 4, 2022.

DOI: https://doi.org/10.2105/AJPH.2022.307147

CONTRIBUTORS

A. D. Rosen prepared the first draft of the article. A. D. Rosen and I. Howerton performed data analysis. E. U. Kantrim, A. H. Chang, A. Nguyen, and E. H. Thomas served as program leads. All authors contributed to program implementation and drafting and revising the article and reviewed and approved the final version of the article.

ACKNOWLEDGMENTS

Housing for Health (HFH) COVID-19 response teams were funded via grants awarded to the Los Angeles County Department of Public Health (ELC Enhancing Detection: 6 NU50CK000498-01-09 and ELC Enhancing Detection Expansion: 6 NU50CK000498-02-04; as supplemental funds for CK19-1904: ELC Enhancing Detection through Coronavirus Response and Relief).

The authors would like to acknowledge the HFH COVID-19 response team, whose dedication to developing meaningful, dignified, and innovative approaches to health care for unhoused people made this work possible. The authors wish to thank their governmental, academic, and community partners, including the Los Angeles County Department of Public Health, for the funding, vaccines, technical support, and collaboration used in this project.

CONFLICTS OF INTEREST

The authors have no conflicts of interest to declare.

HUMAN PARTICIPANT PROJECTION

Institutional review board (IRB) approval was not required for program implementation. Quality improvement studies were determined to be exempt from IRB oversight by the University of California, Los Angeles IRB.

REFERENCES

1. Spicker P. Social Work and Self-determination. *Br J Soc Work*. 1990;20(3):221–236.
2. Willer B, Corrigan JD. Whatever it takes: a model for community-based services. *Brain Inj*. 1994; 8(7):647–659. https://doi.org/10.3109/02699059409151017
3. Shover CL, Rosen A, Mata J, et al. Engaging same-day peer ambassadors to increase coronavirus disease 2019 vaccination among people experiencing unsheltered homelessness in Los Angeles County: a hybrid feasibility–evaluation study. *J Infect Dis*. 2022;226(suppl 3):S346–S352. https://doi.org/10.1093/infdis/jiac291
4. Leifheit KM, Chaisson LH, Medina JA, Wahbi RN, Shover CL. Elevated mortality among people experiencing homelessness with COVID-19. *Open Forum Infect Dis*. 2021;8(7):ofab301. https://doi.org/10.1093/ofid/ofab301
5. Feldman BJ, Kim JS, Mosqueda L, et al. From the hospital to the streets: bringing care to the unsheltered homeless in Los Angeles. *Healthc (Amst)*. 2021;9(3):100557. https://doi.org/10.1016/j.hjdsi.2021.100557
6. Knight KR, Duke MR, Carey CA, et al. COVID-19 testing and vaccine acceptability among homeless-experienced adults: qualitative data from two samples. *J Gen Intern Med*. 2022; 37(4):823–829. https://doi.org/10.1007/s11606-021-07161-1

7. Crawford K. Evaluating Trauma-Informed Care Practices in an Interdisciplinary Homeless Service Collaboration. *J Evidence-Based Soc Work.* 2022; 19(2):212–227.
8. Rosen AD, Beltran J, Thomas E, et al. COVID-19 vaccine acceptability and financial incentives among unhoused people in Los Angeles County: a three-stage field survey. *J Urban Health.* 2022; 99(3):594–602. https://doi.org/10.1007/s11524-022-00659-x
9. Los Angeles Homeless Services Authority. 2020 Greater Los Angeles homeless count results. June 12, 2020. Available at: https://www.lahsa.org/news?article=726-2020-greater-los-angeles-homeless-count-results. Accessed February 28, 2022.
10. County of Los Angeles Public Health. Deaths among people experiencing homelessness. February 18, 2022. Available at: http://www.publichealth.lacounty.gov/phcommon/public/media/mediapubhpdetail.cfm?prid=3697. Accessed October 20, 2022.
11. Rogers JH, Link AC, McCulloch D, et al. Characteristics of COVID-19 in homeless shelters: a community-based surveillance study. *Ann Intern Med.* 2021;174(1):42–49. https://doi.org/10.7326/M20-3799
12. County of Los Angeles Public Health. COVID-19 dashboard: locations and demographics. October 20, 2022. Available at: http://publichealth.lacounty.gov/media/Coronavirus/locations.htm. Accessed February 28, 2022.

New Frameworks for Engaging Communities to Confront HIV, COVID-19, and Climate Change Health Inequities

Jonathan I. Levy, ScD, and Lisa Bowleg, PhD, MA

ABOUT THE AUTHORS

Jonathan I. Levy is with the Department of Environmental Health, Boston University School of Public Health, Boston, MA. Lisa Bowleg is with the Department of Psychological and Brain Sciences, The George Washington University, Washington, DC.

See also Alang and Blackstock, p. 194, Cole et al., p. 185, Ferguson, p. 182, p. 175, Mendéz and Zuñiga p. 177, Razum and Wandschneider, p. 133, and Riley, p. 179.

Climate change, HIV, and COVID-19 are complex global health challenges with inequitable impacts both within and between countries. Although the inequities have been widely acknowledged for some time, numerous factors have made it difficult to make headway in reducing or eliminating them. These factors include structural racism and other forms of discrimination against racial/ethnic minority and low- or no-income populations that lead to differential exposures and differential access to health care. Two articles in the current issue of *AJPH* propose new frameworks that emphasize the importance of empowering communities marginalized by intersecting systems of oppression as the key to addressing inequities. Comparing the articles' proposed frameworks provides some insight into strategies to confront inequities across the field of public health.

Cole et al. (p. 185) propose a typology of health equity–focused community-based climate action, whereby the two key dimensions by which community-based climate action can be evaluated are the extent of community agency and the degree to which power relationships are transformed. At one extreme is a model of quasiparticipation, in which community members can voice their concerns but have no real power to influence decisions and no efforts are made to build community agency. At the other extreme is a model of transformative action, in which decision-making processes are inclusive and there are sustained efforts to empower communities and ensure that they can truly influence decisions. Of the 48 community-based climate action examples the authors review, only 12 fit into the category of transformative action. Examples of transformative action typically include explicit attempts to build community capacity while changing the structure of advisory committees to include community members and allow them to have real decision-making authority.

Similarly, Alang and Blackstock (p. 194) propose a health justice framework that emphasizes the redistribution of power and resources to center the needs of communities and populations that have historically been marginalized, considering both HIV and COVID-19. Using an intersectionality lens that acknowledges race, gender, class, sexuality, and other dimensions, the authors move beyond previously proposed frameworks to explicitly acknowledge that inequities in outcomes arise because of the combined influence of systems, structures, and institutions on health and well-being. Their recommendations include redistributing resources to go beyond an individual choice model that perpetuates structural inequities, using mandates and regulations to redistribute power, and ensuring that the most affected communities are centered during policy development. The authors also reinforce the importance of evaluating the multidimensional effects of policies across systems; beneficial interventions could exacerbate inequities because of differential access to the interventions, or measures used to tackle one form of inequity (e.g., virtual school to reduce inequitable COVID-19 risk) could create another form of inequity (e.g., learning outcomes).

This observation creates a bridge between the two articles: what types of systems and structures would be needed to simultaneously address inequities in climate change, COVID-19, HIV, and other major public health issues? Although this is a daunting challenge, the conceptual frameworks of both articles provide insight into two elements that could be transformational.

First, top-down models in which communities or populations that have been historically marginalized are not given the power to lead and influence decisions will invariably perpetuate inequities. This type of shift in power dynamics

AJPH February 2023, Vol 113, No. 2

often requires policy changes that mandate the representation of affected communities and populations on key advisory committees or in other decision-making bodies, where these committees have real authority and the community members have genuine input and power. Alang and Blackstock give the example of requirements for obtaining part A funds from the Ryan White Program that include demonstrated participation of people living with HIV. Cole et al. give the example of the Oakland Climate Action Coalition, in which city agencies granted community members not just inclusion on advisory committees but also real decision-making authority. These and other examples can be broadened to include other contexts. To formally consider intersections among a range of stressors, mandated representation and associated empowerment should happen in programs targeting individual stressors and programs addressing upstream factors.

Second, many health inequities stem from factors such as systemic and structural racism that lead to both differential access to resources (e.g., the ability to afford medications or nonpharmaceutical interventions) and differential exposures to stressors (e.g., increased exposure to heat related to structural discrimination that influences housing and the built environment). Although addressing these inequities across the board would be challenging, given political resistance and the sheer scale and scope of the problem, both articles point to the need for policy development that centers equity (partly through the empowerment processes described) and that closes gaps created by unaddressed or unacknowledged structural discrimination (through targeted policy measures).

For example, the 2022 US COVID-19 response largely emphasizes individual choice to obtain vaccines or nonpharmaceutical interventions, a strategy that perpetuates inequities by not acknowledging that structural racism and other systems of oppression create differential ability to work from home, get paid sick leave, afford masks or adequate ventilation and filtration, and so forth.[1] An approach consistent with these conceptual models would formally engage those disproportionately affected by COVID-19 for multiple reasons (e.g., disability status, essential worker status, lack of health insurance) and use their input to craft programs that reduce financial and logistical barriers.

Both articles also intersect with the broader domain of community-based participatory research, in which community members are directly involved in research efforts that will influence their communities, often with a health equity lens.[2] Although neither article formally addresses community-based participatory research, the conceptual framework—which is captured fundamentally by the expression "nothing about us without us"—provides some helpful additional elements. In particular, research in communities will not be as successful in effectuating change unless the community has a leadership role in determining the research question, contributing to the data collection, and informing the analysis and ultimate interpretation. There are multiple examples of community-based participatory research studies that were able to redistribute power from researchers to community members and were therefore able to have a greater influence on the policy process.[3,4]

The sheer magnitude of health inequities and their disparate impact on historically marginalized communities demand new and unconventional models of community engagement. In proposing new frameworks, these articles flip the script and center the role of community in advancing health equity. Together, these articles offer new pathways to transformational change for the public health community and the key decision-makers charged with protecting community health. AJPH

CORRESPONDENCE

Correspondence should be sent to Jonathan I. Levy, Professor and Chair, Department of Environmental Health, Boston University School of Public Health, 715 Albany St T4W, Boston, MA 02118 (e-mail: jonlevy@bu.edu). Reprints can be ordered at http://www.ajph.org by clicking the "Reprints" link.

PUBLICATION INFORMATION

Full Citation: Levy JI, Bowleg L. New frameworks for engaging communities to confront HIV, COVID-19, and climate change health inequities. *Am J Public Health*. 2023;113(2):175–176.

Acceptance Date: November 20, 2022.

DOI: https://doi.org/10.2105/AJPH.2022.307188

CONTRIBUTORS

J. I. Levy and L. Bowleg jointly prepared the editorial and made equal contributions to its content.

CONFLICTS OF INTEREST

We have no potential or actual conflicts of interest to declare.

REFERENCES

1. Selden TM, Berdahl TA. COVID-19 and racial/ethnic disparities in health risk, employment, and household composition. *Health Aff (Millwood)*. 2020;39(9): 1624–1632. https://doi.org/10.1377/hlthaff.2020.00897
2. Ward M, Schulz AJ, Israel BA, Rice K, Martenies SE, Markarian E. A conceptual framework for evaluating health equity promotion within community-based participatory research partnerships. *Eval Program Plann*. 2018;70:25–34. https://doi.org/10.1016/j.evalprogplan.2018.04.014
3. Gonzalez PA, Minkler M, Garcia AP, et al. Community-based participatory research and policy advocacy to reduce diesel exposure in West Oakland, California. *Am J Public Health*. 2011;101(suppl 1): S166–S175. https://doi.org/10.2105/AJPH.2010.196204
4. Sprague Martinez L, Dimitri N, Ron S, et al. Two communities, one highway and the fight for clean air: the role of political history in shaping community engagement and environmental health research translation. *BMC Public Health*. 2020;20(1):1690. https://doi.org/10.1186/s12889-020-09751-w

Understanding Challenges to Health Equity in Climate Action and Land Use Planning

Michael Méndez, PhD, MCP, and Michelle E. Zuñiga, PhD

ABOUT THE AUTHORS

Michael Méndez is with the Department of Urban Planning and Public Policy, University of California, Irvine. Michelle E. Zuñiga is with the Department of Geography and Earth Sciences, University of North Carolina, Charlotte.

See also Cole et al., p. 185, Ferguson, p. 182, Levy and Bowleg, p. 175, Razum and Wandschneider, p. 133, and Riley, p. 179.

Cole et al. (p. 185 in this issue of *AJPH*) argue that health equity is crucial to addressing the human health consequences of climate change. They underscore how effective climate action requires meaningful public engagement processes focused on increasing community capacity and the power to reduce health disparities in marginalized neighborhoods. Such findings are consistent with Méndez's[1] study of the challenges of incorporating health equity into local climate action plans. That research focused on how California's cities with high levels of pollution and social vulnerability address climate change and public health. In general, the findings showed that in these cities, climate action planning and work on public health were occurring in a parallel manner rather than through an integrated approach. The study, moreover, highlighted the need to develop stronger partnerships with community-based organizations for linking climate action planning with public health.

Cole et al., accordingly, in their recent study of 48 community-based climate actions, reference Arnstein's "Ladder of Citizen Participation"[2] and explore how some of the climate actions offered the illusion of participation without any meaningful resident engagement. Furthermore, many of these climate actions failed to provide opportunities for power building: the empowerment of marginalized communities with the voice, capacity, and authority to determine how and what methods are needed to reduce health disparities through climate action measures.

Our forthcoming research takes a similar approach. We analyzed the tensions stakeholders (i.e., government, community, and consultants) have in implementing a new California law (Senate Bill 1000) that requires environmental justice considerations (bit.ly/3FsN7Zh; bit.ly/3iJL5vM) to be included in local land use plans (i.e., general plans). Our analysis of 37 city and county general plans in localities determined by the state to have high levels of environmental injustice shows that they had minimal resources to carry out measures and engage in substantive community engagement.[3] However, one approach to help overcome this challenge is urban planners' use of a strong public health framing.

Three of 37 jurisdictions in our study referred to a previous health strategy (i.e., chapter or element) in their general plans as an important precursor for environmental justice considerations. These localities began their outreach with a broad discussion on health as a method for residents to understand and relate contextually to environmental justice (bit.ly/3Bhdyjc; bit.ly/3h3U1vE). The health chapter helped urban planners understand the disparities and detail them in the general plan. This contextual analysis of existing conditions and identification of vulnerable populations also served as a guide for community outreach. Similarly, local public health departments assisted urban planners to better understand community and environmental health needs. We found that four jurisdictions had partnered with them. These partnerships were instrumental in guiding community engagement and acquiring, sharing, and analyzing data, as well as developing goals and policies related to environmental justice.

One key example is the City of Los Angeles, California, which in 2021 established the Climate Emergency Mobilization Office. The office has made interdepartmental policy recommendations in partnership with community groups, centering environmental justice considerations related to climate change, disasters, and land use. These recommendations will be included in the city's next general plan update. In particular, the office is promoting a strong focus on health and climate change and working with community-based health and governmental experts on proposed measures and proposals. This approach is consistent with the typology of "transformative action" in health equity processes in Cole et al. The city is helping build community power through advisory boards and the substantive integration of local knowledge in key planning documents. It provides a more egalitarian process for inclusive decision-making.[4] Similarly, we found that localities that established environmental justice advisory committees through transformative actions reported having more robust conversations about racial and environmental health inequities and were able to better develop substantive environmental justice policies in their general plans.[5]

In sum, Cole et al. provide a strong foundation to understand effective methods for community power building and engagement processes to reduce health disparities through climate action measures. However, there is still much to learn from how local governments, urban planners, and community groups have navigated health equity implementation and how jurisdictions with varying landscapes and political contexts can establish policies that will reduce health disparities and mitigate the harms of our changing climate.[6,7] As the authors acknowledge, more in-depth research focused on case studies, stakeholder interviews, and other qualitative data are needed. Nonetheless, their research is an important step forward in the development of more integrative and transformative health equity and climate action planning efforts. AJPH

CORRESPONDENCE

Correspondence should be sent to Michael Méndez, MCP, PhD, University of California, Irvine, Department of Urban Planning and Public Policy, 300 Social Ecology I, Irvine, CA 92697-7075 (e-mail: mamende6@uci.edu). Reprints can be ordered at http://www.ajph.org by clicking the "Reprints" link.

PUBLICATION INFORMATION

Full Citation: Méndez M, Zuñiga ME. Understanding challenges to health equity in climate action and land use planning. *Am J Public Health*. 2023;113(2): 177–178.

Acceptance Date: November 22, 2022.

DOI: https://doi.org/10.2105/AJPH.2022.307189

CONTRIBUTORS

M. Méndez supervised the editorial. Both authors wrote, edited, and conceptualized the editorial.

CONFLICTS OF INTEREST

The authors have no conflicts of interest to declare.

REFERENCES

1. Méndez MA. Assessing local climate action plans for public health co-benefits in environmental justice communities. *Local Environ*. 2015;20(6):637–663. https://doi.org/10.1080/13549839.2015.1038227
2. Arnstein SR. A ladder of citizen participation. *J Am Plann Assoc*. 1969;35(4):216–224. https://doi.org/10.1080/01944366908977225
3. Méndez M. The reflective practitioner in the context of racial and environmental justice. *Plann Theory Pract*. 2022;23(3):425–458. https://doi.org/10.1080/14649357.2022.2082710
4. Rifkin SB. A framework linking community empowerment and health equity: it is a matter of CHOICE. *J Health Popul Nutr*. 2003;21(3):168–180.
5. Tritter JQ, McCallum A. The snakes and ladders of user involvement: moving beyond Arnstein. *Health Policy*. 2006;76(2):156–168. https://doi.org/10.1016/j.healthpol.2005.05.008
6. Méndez M. *Climate Change From the Streets: How Conflict and Collaboration Strengthen the Environmental Justice Movement*. New Haven, CT: Yale University Press; 2020.
7. Goldsmith L, Raditz V, Méndez M. Queer and present danger: understanding the disparate impacts of disasters on LGBTQ+ communities. *Disasters*. 2022; 46(4):946–973. https://doi.org/10.1111/disa.12509

Redefining the Quest for Health Equity in the Era of Climate Crisis

Alicia R. Riley, PhD, MPH, MA

ABOUT THE AUTHOR

Alicia R. Riley is with the Department of Sociology, University of California Santa Cruz.

See also Cole et al., p. 185, Ferguson, p. 182, Levy and Bowleg, p. 175, Mendéz and Zuñiga p. 177, and Razum and Wandschneider, p. 133.

Public health has a problem: despite widespread commitments to "advance health equity," few could specify exactly what health equity would look like in an ideal world, much less in the face of the climate crisis. We have tended to define health equity by what it is not—by evidence of health inequities. As such, health equity itself has remained an intangible goal—easy to align with as a value, much harder to specify or make happen in practice. However, we find ourselves in a quickening climate crisis that makes calls to "advance health equity" feel simultaneously more urgent and more utopian. For health equity to be more than just a slogan going forward, public health must define a process for achieving and sustaining health equity.

A study by Cole et al. (p. 185) takes up the challenge of defining the process to advance health equity in the climate crisis era. The authors ask two questions: what does health equity in community-based climate action look like in practice, and how should public health scholars and practitioners assess progress and gaps? In response, they propose a novel typology that can guide scholars and practitioners in pursuing not just the concept of health equity but also the ongoing practice of health equity. The typology centers two axes of progress toward climate-relevant health equity: community agency and community power. Cole et al. argue that to mitigate health inequities stemming from the climate crisis, the pursuit of health equity must focus on increasing community agency and transforming power.

Cole et al.'s typology has several strengths. First, it is practical. Too often, scholarship on health equity is bogged down by flowery language and ill-defined idealism. Instead, Cole et al.'s two-by-two typology offers a concrete framework that prioritizes specific kinds of action. Second, Cole et al.'s typology views health equity as a process rather than a destination. The typology is designed to assess progress, diagnose gaps, and facilitate course corrections. In this way, it is a realistic tool for community organizations or funding agencies to incorporate into their existing regular assessments. Third, it is easy to imagine the Cole et al. typology being applied to multiple domains of public health practice. While Cole et al.'s typology was developed specifically to assess actions contributing to health equity in climate action, the typology uses general concepts (inclusion, quasi-participation, capacity building, and transformative action) that are easily identifiable in a wide range of community-based actions.

However, the usefulness of Cole et al.'s typology in practice depends on the extent to which scholars and practitioners agree with how Cole et al. conceptualize health equity itself. In the article, Cole et al. explain that under their vision for health equity, reducing health disparities is essential but also insufficient. They emphasize that health equity is "also a process of empowering previously marginalized communities with the voice, capacity, power, and authority to set their own health priorities and to determine how those priorities are addressed" (p. 186). They also acknowledge that how we define what equity-promoting initiatives look like has implications for practice. Indeed, this is where there is room for further dialogue about our collective vision for health equity and how this may need to evolve in the era of the climate crisis.

REDISTRIBUTING POWER AND RESOURCES

Before the climate crisis era, the idea of redistributing health to achieve health equity seemed taboo and even unethical. Still today, public health scholars remain far more interested in countering the unfair disadvantages in health than in countering the unfair advantages. For the most part, this makes sense, because health is a special good; there is a moral imperative to meet health needs.[1,2] Thus, it can seem wrong to aim to reduce health-promoting resources, such as money, prestige, and power, under any circumstances, even if those reductions would bring health equity into balance. However, being that health advantages are created through the same unfair

AJPH February 2023, Vol 113, No. 2

processes that create health disadvantages, we may be slowing our progress toward health equity by ignoring one side of the distribution. Sociologists Link and García refer to this tendency for researchers to disregard the actions of advantaged groups that generate health inequities as health-inequality diversions.[3] Diversions distract from the necessary work of interrogating the White supremacist and exploitative ideologies that obscure and justify the inequitable distribution of resources.[4]

The climate crisis decisively clarifies that the work to advance health equity must transform resources on the side of the already powerful. The necessary redistribution of resources involves not just a building up on the low side of the distribution but also a reining in on the high side; it requires not just climate change adaptation in impacted communities but also regulations to halt the progression of global warming. Through policy change, consumer pressure, and community organizing, the possibility of "buying" health or buying one's way out of the health threats of climate change must be limited. Of course, the quest for health equity should not occur through a leveling down of health. But the path surely involves policy and cultural shifts to curb resource overconsumption among advantaged groups. The question then becomes not whether policies should redistribute health-promoting resources but how resource redistribution can be achieved in a way that is ethical and sustainable.

The work to prevent and undo unfair resource advantages is not explicit in Cole et al.'s proposed typology, which focuses on "engagement of vulnerable and marginalized populations" (p. 185). As such, there is a risk that practitioners who apply the typology will focus on empowering marginalized communities without attention to the powerful interests that maintain and profit from that marginalization. However, the goal of transformative action that Cole et al. advocate in their article is key to holding powerful actors accountable to facilitate resource redistribution. Community organizing builds the power necessary to counterbalance state and corporate agendas that undermine health equity.

MAXIMIZING PLANETARY HEALTH

Living in the climate crisis era also challenges us to redefine what it means to "maximize" health. The mainstream vision for health equity anchors its definition of maximal health on the level of health enjoyed by the most advantaged group. Under this vision, health equity is achieved when the disadvantaged parts of the distribution are brought up to the level of health enjoyed by the advantaged parts. The problem with this vision is that it is narrowly focused on maximizing individual health, often at the expense of planetary health. With current extremes of global income inequality, a vision for health equity modeled on the levels of resource consumption of the most advantaged risks contributing to the depletion of the Earth's ecosystems and natural resources. This is because now, more than ever, maximizing consumption of resources does not maximize health. Herein lies a challenge but also an opportunity.

Public health as a field has yet to commit to an alternative path to health equity that involves less resource consumption, less accumulation, less convenience, and less exploitation of natural resources and human labor. The current moment calls us to explore planetary-level measures of health and to study the interconnectedness of planetary health and individual health. For nearly 15 years, there have been isolated calls to consider health equity on a planetary scale.[5] If we are to achieve health equity amid recurrent climate emergencies, we must now take seriously the work of resource use reduction, resource redistribution, resource renewal, and sustainable systems of food and urban development. This means that we need tangible examples of what working toward health equity looks like in practice, which Cole et al. provide in their article, but we also need our vision for health equity to incorporate planetary health. Cole et al.'s typology is useful for thinking about health equity in individual and community health, but it does not explicitly resolve conflicts that may emerge when efforts to maximize health equity in individual health occur at the expense of planetary health equity. The community-based climate actions featured in the analysis by Cole et al. have a local lens. Similar research needs to be done to analyze the process of working toward health equity on a planetary scale.

The article by Cole et al. invites public health scholars and practitioners to specify what we mean when we say, "advance health equity," how we will measure progress, and how we will apply our work to the greatest challenge of our era: the climate crisis. They offer a vision that emphasizes bottom-up work to build community agency and power. Here, I argue that the process to advance health equity in the climate crisis era must also include steps to redistribute power and resources and must trade the goal of maximizing individual health for the goal of maximizing planetary health. Others may have different views of successful advancement of health equity. By giving us something to react to, Cole et al. push us to make the work to advance health equity real. AJPH

CORRESPONDENCE

Correspondence should be sent to Alicia R. Riley, PhD, MPH, MA, Assistant Professor of Sociology and Core Faculty in Global and Community Health, University of California, Santa Cruz, 1156 High St, Santa Cruz, CA 95064 (e-mail: alicia.riley@ucsc.edu). Reprints can be ordered at https://ajph.org by clicking the "Reprints" link.

PUBLICATION INFORMATION

Full Citation: Riley AR. Redefining the quest for health equity in the era of climate crisis. *Am J Public Health*. 2023;113(2):179–181.

Acceptance Date: November 22, 2022.

DOI: https://doi.org/10.2105/AJPH.2022.307187

CONFLICTS OF INTEREST

The author reports no conflicts of interest.

REFERENCES

1. Daniels N. *Just Health: Meeting Health Needs Fairly*. New York, NY: Cambridge University Press; 2007. https://doi.org/10.1017/CBO9780511809514
2. Epstein RA. Why is health care special? *Univ Kans Law Rev*. 1992;40:307–324.
3. Link BG, García SJ. Diversions: how the underrepresentation of research on advantaged groups leaves explanations for health inequalities incomplete. *J Health Soc Behav*. 2021;62(3):334–349. https://doi.org/10.1177/00221465211028152
4. García SJ, Trummel T, Cornejo M, et al. Immigrant health inequities: exposing diversions and White supremacy. *Soc Sci*. 2021;10(9):341. https://doi.org/10.3390/socsci10090341
5. Friel S, Marmot M, McMichael AJ, Kjellstrom T, Vågerö D. Global health equity and climate stabilisation: a common agenda. *Lancet*. 2008;372(9650):1677–1683. https://doi.org/10.1016/S0140-6736(08)61692-X

Health Justice in the Context of Health and Human Rights

Laura Ferguson, PhD

ABOUT THE AUTHOR

Laura Ferguson is with the Institute on Inequalities in Global Health, University of Southern California, Los Angeles.

See also Alang and Blackstock, p. 194, Cole et al., p. 185, Levy and Bowleg, p. 175, Mendéz and Zuñiga, p. 177, Razum and Wandschneider, p. 133, and Riley, p. 179.

In their analytic essay "Health Justice: A Framework for Mitigating the Impacts of HIV and COVID-19 on Disproportionately Affected Communities" (p. 194), Alang and Blackstock propose a health justice framework for understanding and responding to the inequalities exposed and exacerbated by recent pandemics including HIV and COVID-19. Redressing inequitable distributions of power and resources is seen as a pathway toward liberation and advancement of traditionally oppressed communities, and a range of structural interventions are proposed for advancing this work.

This framework, specific to HIV and COVID-19, resonates with the previous work of Benfer et al. on health justice more broadly as well as their recent COVID-19–specific analyses.[1,2] Indeed, although health justice has been variably defined, the notion of redistribution of power and resources is often central.[3–5] Aligned with previous conceptualizations of health justice, Alang and Blackstock focus on the specificities regarding two recent pandemics and how responses to them might be strengthened.

Alang and Blackstock's conceptualization also speaks to many of the key principles of work at the intersection of health and human rights. Although there is a longer history of work at the intersection of women's health and human rights, it was in the context of HIV that the relationships between health and human rights were first systematically explored.

Jonathan Mann was a pioneer of health and human rights. Trained as a medical doctor and epidemiologist, he spearheaded the first global strategy on HIV while leading the World Health Organization's Global Program on AIDS. He then moved into academia, where he explored how vulnerability to HIV was intertwined with the lack of realization of human rights, which laid the groundwork for developing the health and human rights framework.[6]

Mann and colleagues posited three important relationships between health and human rights: (1) health policies, programs, and practices affect (positively and negatively) human rights; (2) violations of human rights have important health effects; and (3) an inextricable link exists between the promotion and protection of health and the promotion and protection of human rights and dignity.[7] Although initially designed in relation to HIV, this framework was later expanded to be relevant to health more broadly.

The three relationships between health and human rights identified in Mann and colleagues' early work can be seen in Alang and Blackstock's essay on health justice. The authors identified shortfalls in policies, programs, and practices in response to HIV and COVID-19 that have had a negative impact on human rights. Such shortfalls include the initial politically motivated nonresponse by governments that fueled not only disease spread but also discrimination against the marginalized populations initially hit hardest by each pandemic.

Resistance to policies such as Medicare for All can be seen as a violation of the right to health, which encompasses the notion of affordability of health services for everyone. As Alang and Blackstock note, there have been gross inequities in access to pandemic prevention and treatment interventions. These inequities can be seen as violations of the rights to health, to equality and nondiscrimination, and to the enjoyment of the benefits of scientific progress. It cannot be assumed that if a technology exists, it is equally available to all. Historical distrust of the medical system, lack of access to information, cost, and health provider bias all play important roles in determining the true accessibility and acceptability of these interventions.

The inextricable link between the promotion and protection of both health and human rights comes to the fore in the lack of attention to structural determinants in pandemic responses. That racially minoritized groups bear a disproportionate COVID-19 burden stems, as the authors note, from centuries of structural racism that have deliberately marginalized these populations. The lack of attention to these systemic and structural drivers of vulnerability in pandemic responses illustrates a critical shortcoming. If we rely on the indivisibility and interrelatedness of human rights—that no right can be considered alone and that the realization of rights is mutually interdependent—it is clear that the promotion and protection of, in this case, the rights to nondiscrimination and to health must be jointly addressed.

The structural interventions proposed also align with this early conceptualization of health and human rights. Human rights, by design, challenge power imbalances. By requiring that rather than treating everyone the same, additional efforts be made to reach and elevate the most marginalized and discriminated against, human rights incorporate the notion of redistributive justice, expressed by Alang and Blackstock as the need to "ensure access to and redistribution of resources." Linking to the legal basis of the health and human rights framework, the authors also call for the "introduction of mandates and enforcement of regulations that redistribute power" and for "legislation that guarantees support for people with long-haul COVID-19." Along with evaluations of "intersecting and multidimensional effects of policies across systems," this draws attention to accountability, which is considered central to work at the intersection of health and human rights; the difference between laws and policies on paper and "on the streets" has been frequently highlighted.[8,9]

We need to know what works and what does not work; we also need to know who is fulfilling their obligations in the context of health and human rights and who is not. Central to all of this, and reflecting the right to participation, is the need to "center the experiences of the most impacted communities in policy development." Taken together, the structural interventions proposed in Alang and Blackstock's essay seek to ensure that health policies, programs, and actions support human rights, reduce violations of human rights that affect health, and support the mutual promotion and protection of health and rights.

In recent years, scholars and implementers have adopted "rights-based approaches to health" as a way of operationalizing human rights within health interventions. Initial conceptions of rights-based approaches to health were often disease specific, but over time the need to apply them to health more broadly became clear. They now encompass a widely accepted set of human rights and rights principles: attention to the legal and policy environment; participation; equality and nondiscrimination; the availability, accessibility, acceptability, and quality of services; and accountability.[10] Such rights-based approaches to health require systematic and rigorous attention to many of the same issues as Alang and Blackstock's health justice framework. It will be interesting to see whether there is further development of this health justice framework beyond its current specificity to pandemics, a trajectory that many initially disease-specific models have taken.

Mann and colleagues' initial conceptualization of health and human rights remains as relevant today in the context of COVID-19 as it was in the context of HIV. Furthermore, more recent work has built from this foundation to strengthen the evidence of the value of work at the intersection of health and human rights. There is, today, more recognition of historical legacies of marginalization and discrimination that negatively affect health and some initial acceptance that societal divisions are as important to consider in pandemic responses as biomedical vulnerability to disease. Yet, what is still missing is large-scale action to tackle these deep-rooted, complex problems. Pandemic preparedness remains focused on biomedical capacity rather than tackling the structures and systems that permeate inequality and injustice and that will continue to disadvantage specific populations in any future pandemic.

Health justice can usefully be grounded in human rights. Underpinned by international law, human rights provide a framework for systematic consideration of the wide range of structural determinants of health inequities alongside the legal obligations of governments to ensure that these inequities are addressed. The strong history of community organizing and grassroots activism among the human rights community might indeed be leveraged to push for government action and accountability at the local, state, and national levels. AJPH

CORRESPONDENCE

Correspondence should be sent to Laura Ferguson, PhD, Soto Street Building, 318H, 1845 North Soto St, MC 9239, Los Angeles, CA 90089-9239 (e-mail: laura.ferguson@med.usc.edu). Reprints can be ordered at http://www.ajph.org by clicking the "Reprints" link.

PUBLICATION INFORMATION

Full Citation: Ferguson L. Health justice in the context of health and human rights. *Am J Public Health*. 2023;113(2):182–184.

Acceptance Date: November 29, 2022.

DOI: https://doi.org/10.2105/AJPH.2022.307184

CONFLICTS OF INTEREST

The author has no conflicts of interest to declare.

REFERENCES

1. Benfer EA. Health justice: a framework (and call to action) for the elimination of health inequity and social justice. *Am Univ Law Rev.* 2015;65: 275–351.
2. Benfer EA, Mohapatra S, Wiley LF, Yearby R. Health justice strategies to combat the pandemic: eliminating discrimination, poverty, and health disparities during and after COVID-19. *Yale J Health Policy Law Ethics.* 2020;19(3):122–171.
3. Harris AP, Pamukcu A. The civil rights of health: a new approach to challenging structural inequality. *UCLA Law Rev.* 2020;67:758–832.
4. Makhlouf MD. Health Justice for Immigrants. Available at: https://www.immigrationresearch.org/system/files/Health_Justice.pdf. Accessed November 20, 2022.
5. Wiley LF. From patient rights to health justice: securing the public's interest in affordable, high-quality health care. *Cardozo Law Rev.* 2015;37: 833–889.
6. Tarantola D, Gruskin S, Brown TM, Fee E. Jonathan Mann. *Am J Public Health.* 2006;96(11):1942–1943. https://doi.org/10.2105/AJPH.2006.098079
7. Mann JM, Gostin L, Gruskin S, Brennan T, Lazzarini Z, Fineberg HV. Health and human rights. *Health Hum Rights.* 1994;1(1):6–23.
8. Ferguson L, Jardell W, Lambert-Peck M, et al. Mind the gap: understanding differences between sexual and reproductive health-related legal frameworks on paper and in practice. *Front Glob Womens Health.* 2022;3:838976. https://doi.org/10.3389%2Ffgwh.2022.838976
9. Poncz E. Rethinking child advocacy after Roper v. Simmons: kids are just different and kids are like adults advocacy strategies. *Cardozo Public Law Policy Ethics J.* 2008;6(273):292–293.
10. Gruskin S, Bogecho D, Ferguson L. 'Rights-based approaches' to health policies and programs: articulations, ambiguities, and assessment. *J Public Health Policy.* 2010;31(2):129–145. https://doi.org/10.1057/jphp.2010.7

Advancing Health Equity in Community-Based Climate Action: From Concept to Practice

Brian L. Cole, DrPH, Irish Del Rosario, MPH, Astrid Hendricks, PhD, and David P. Eisenman, MD, MSHS

See also Ferguson, p. 182, Levy and Bowleg, p. 175, Mendéz and Zuñiga p. 177, Razum and Wandschneider, p. 133, and Riley, p. 179.

Despite broad agreement that prioritizing health equity is critical to minimizing the health impacts of climate change, there is a lack of clarity about what advancing health equity means in practice. More than reducing health disparities; it also implies engaging and empowering marginalized communities.

We propose a typology of health equity processes, focused on building community agency and power, and then apply it to a nonrepresentative, purposive sample of 48 community-based climate actions (CBCAs) selected from lists of projects funded by foundations and state climate programs and from other sources. All CBCAs were in the United States, community-based, active since 2015 or more recently, engaged in climate mitigation or adaptation, and stated health equity aims. Two team members reviewed project reports to assess the engagement of vulnerable and marginalized populations, agency-building, and transformation of community power relationships.

Although 33 CBCAs reported efforts to build community agency, only 19 reported efforts to increase community power. City-led CBCAs showed less emphasis on agency-building and power transformation. This typology can support efforts to advance health equity by providing concrete indicators to diagnose gaps and track progress. (*Am J Public Health*. 2023;113(2):185–193. https://doi.org/10.2105/AJPH.2022.307143)

AJPH February 2023, Vol 113, No. 2

Climate change, the greatest public health issue of our time,[1] will cause unprecedented disruption to the physical, biological, and social systems that support human life. Impoverished and socially marginalized populations with the least adaptive resources[2–4] will likely experience the most severe impacts, thus widening existing health disparities.[2,4–6] Reducing health and other inequities can decrease vulnerability to climate-related health risks, and increase community capacity to effectively respond and recover from climate-related threats, such as vector-borne disease, crop failure, floods, and drought.[7] Conversely, climate actions such as reducing greenhouse gas emissions and urban greening can yield health cobenefits for these vulnerable groups.[8,9]

Advancing health equity is critical to both improving population health overall[10] and addressing the health impacts of climate change. Although public health practitioners may share a broad consensus about the importance of addressing health equity, definitions of "health equity" are often vague and inconsistent.[11] Even less clear is how health equity is operationalized in interventions.[12,13] A clear definition of health equity can help guide community initiatives to maximize health equity objectives, articulate to stakeholders and funders how these objectives will be attained, identify threats, and suggest metrics for measuring progress.

With the aim of providing guidance on measuring and supporting health equity efforts in climate action, we identify specific activities that advance health equity at the community level, drawing on theories of community participation, organizing, and empowerment, and propose a typology for assessing health equity efforts in community-based climate action (CBCA). Our goal was not to conduct a systematic survey of practices to advance health equity, but rather to analyze and organize exemplars of the processes that promote health equity across a range of different projects and communities. It is admittedly an outsider perspective on processes that are primarily driven by community insiders.

A Community Focus for Climate Adaptation

This examination of health equity in climate action focuses on local, community-level projects, programs, and policies. Community-level action is particularly important for climate adaptation. Although climate mitigation efforts, such as carbon taxes and phasing out greenhouse gas–emitting electrical power generation, require top-down national- and global-scale action, the success of local climate adaptation efforts to deal with current and anticipated changes in climate hinges on bottom-up engagement of stakeholder communities.[14,15]

Definitions of Health Equity

Reducing health disparities is an essential part of advancing health equity, but it is not enough. Health equity is also a process of empowering previously marginalized communities with the voice, capacity, power, and authority to set their own health priorities and to determine how those priorities are addressed. Braveman et al. put the reduction of health disparities at the center of their definition of health equity, which they defined as "reducing and ultimately eliminating disparities in health and its determinants that adversely affect excluded or marginalized groups."[13] They emphasized, however, that health equity encompasses processes of (1) removing obstacles and increasing opportunities for everyone to be healthier, and (2) ensuring that everyone has a fair and just opportunity to be as healthy as possible.

The World Health Organization's Committee on Social Disparities put an even stronger emphasis on health equity as process, stating that "health equity vitally depends on the empowerment of individuals and groups to represent their needs and interests."[16(p155)] Echoing this emphasis, Susan Rifkin asserted that advancing health equity requires the development of community capabilities and empowerment that enable greater autonomy and agency.[17]

Although empowerment is central to health equity and community engagement, it is also a contested term.[18–21] Sardenberg[18] proposed the term "liberating empowerment" to differentiate transformative empowerment of marginalized groups through collective action from top-down, outsider-led "liberal empowerment" that could be disempowering. Liberating empowerment requires building power with and between the powerless, as well as dismantling the structures through which the powerful maintain power.[18,20,21]

These definitions have implications for practice—what equity-promoting initiatives look like, who is involved, and in what roles. Some definitions emphasize outcomes and are agnostic on how or even if community members have a meaningful role in planning and implementation. Top-down policies and provision of services may improve some health outcomes, particularly around climate mitigation and disaster response, where national and international action is required; however, if advancing health equity in its broadest sense is a goal, then bottom-up community engagement is also essential.

Building Community Agency and Power

Understanding the building blocks of community engagement can help guide strategies to advance health equity and measure their progress, whether part of climate adaptation efforts or other initiatives. Theories of community participation[22–24] and community organizations[25–27] suggest 2 interacting processes that shape community engagement: (1) building of community capacity and agency, and (2) transformation of power relationships. Drawing from Newman and Dale,[28] we define community agency as the ability of a community to chart their own course in identifying and addressing risks to their well-being and visions for their future. Building agency involves an interplay of individual-level and collective transformation with the development of individuals' knowledge, self-awareness, and skills that complement the development of collective potential, such as growing organizations and coalitions.[19]

Power is about who has the authority and means to effect change.[29] Although agency and power are distinct, they complement each other; empowerment requires development of agency within a community,[18,30] whereas building community agency requires power.[28]

A Typology of Community Action for Health Equity

The proposed typology shown in Figure 1 displays examples of community-based climate action operating along these 2 dimensions of agency and power, like the typologies of community planning and organization outlined by Rothman[25] and Stockdale.[31] It is assumed that this typology would be applied to actions involving marginalized and vulnerable populations.

The typology's horizontal axis represents the degree to which actions build agency within the community. Do

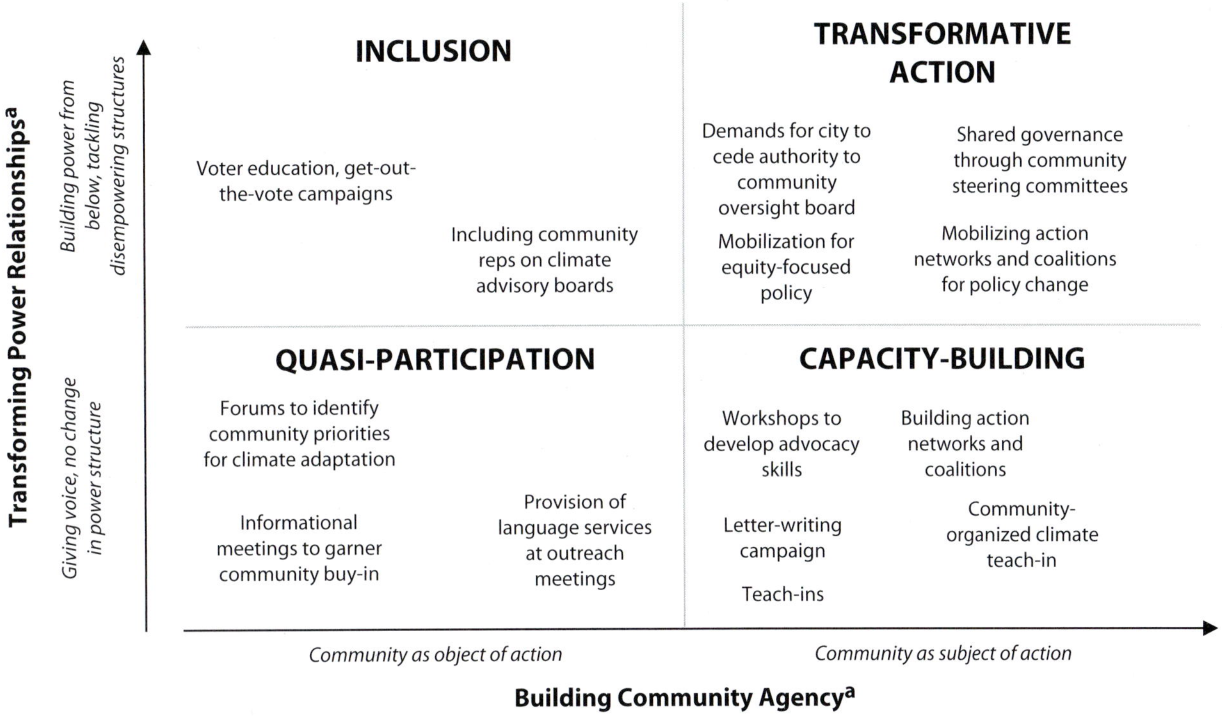

FIGURE 1— Typology of Health Equity–Focused Community-Based Climate Action (CBCA), With Examples of Activities Categorized Across 2 Dimensions of Community Engagement: Building Community Agency and Transforming Power Relationships

[a]All actions in this typology share a focus on working with vulnerable and marginalized populations.

these efforts enable marginalized and vulnerable groups to act more on their own behalf, as the subjects of action? Or do these groups remain the objects of others' actions? The vertical axis differentiates actions based on the degree to which they attempt to change the rules and structures of political power in support of the liberating empowerment of marginalized groups as described by Sardenberg.[18] Actions are differentiated by the question, "Do actions merely aim to transform power structures for more shared decision-making, or do they leave power structures intact?" The interplay suggests 4 categories of health equity–focused community action, which we have labeled quasi-participation, capacity-building, inclusion, and transformative action (Figure 1). Working with marginalized and vulnerable populations is an assumed element for all 4 approaches.

The first of the 4 approaches, quasi-participation, involves engaging communities with little or no effort to build internal community agency or external power, like Stockdale's "traditional planning,"[31] the "tokenism" in Arnstein's Ladder of Participation,[22] and the top-down, department-driven initiatives in Morgan and Lifshay's Ladder of Community Participation for health departments.[32] Officials from public agencies are firmly in charge of planning and implementing climate action. Although community stakeholders are invited to voice their concerns, those in formal positions of power determine the rules for expressing those concerns and whether those concerns are incorporated into policy decisions.

The second approach, capacity-building, includes actions that involve little or no efforts to change power relationships in the community, akin to what Rothman[25] described as "community capacity development" and the "locality development" in Rothman and Stockdale's earlier models.[25,31] In this approach, community members might receive training on how to navigate the corridors of power and give voice to their concerns but not with the aim of changing how decisions are made or who is making them.

Actions in the third quadrant, inclusion, involve some opening in community decision-making processes to marginalized and vulnerable groups but without broad changes in power structures. Although select individuals may be engaged as community representatives, the status quo of top-down decision-making is left largely intact. The scope and breadth of changes in power relationships within this quadrant may vary greatly. Variations of this approach may include either bottom-up advocacy or top-down planning.

The fourth quadrant, transformative action, includes efforts to build community agency while at the same time opening power structures for broader, more inclusive participation in decision-making. These are not just singular, time-limited campaigns but rather sustained efforts to transform access to power and mechanisms of governance.[20]

METHODS

We sought to identify exemplars of CBCAs that could illustrate the 4 models suggested in our typology. We identified 48 CBCAs from 6 sources (Table 1) using a nonrepresentative, purposive sampling approach. Sources included a peer-reviewed journal article[33] on health and environmental justice in climate action plans, a report from the National Association of Climate Resilience Planners,[34] Web sites of philanthropic foundations and California state programs known to the authors to fund community-based health and climate projects, and a Web search using the terms "community-based" + "climate action" + "health equity" + "projects." Inclusion criteria for the sample included (1) US location, (2) being community-based (i.e., engaging community organizations or focused on effecting change in a particular community), (3) stating that climate mitigation or adaptation was a primary goal, and (4) stating health equity or health disparities reduction as a goal. We excluded initiatives for which climate action was a secondary or incidental consideration, such as public health initiatives that included climate-related co-benefits. Although the search specified "projects," we also included any programs and policy initiatives that appeared in the results. We excluded initiatives that had not been at least partially implemented because these had no process information necessary for categorization of their efforts. To keep a consistent focus on local community-based action, we also excluded initiatives that appeared to be implemented solely by government agencies without any element of community engagement, such as construction of flood-control infrastructure.

Sampled CBCAs were reviewed and coded by 2 of the authors. Reports of the sampled CBCAs were first reviewed to verify that they met all the inclusion criteria and to ascertain what types of activities were under way and planned for each of the projects. Each CBCA was then examined to identify actions affecting community agency and power relationships, which were then categorized in the typology shown in Figure 1. We did not attempt to review all the activities that a given organization might be undertaking, only those cited in reports and organization Web sites as being directly part of the CBCA. As such, classifications of CBCAs should be seen as classification of initiatives, not necessarily classification of entire organizations.

RESULTS

A description of the 48 CBCAs included in the sample is provided in Table A (available as a supplement to the online

TABLE 1— Number of Community-Based Climate Actions Reviewed, by Source of Report

Primary Source	Type of Source	Count
Kresge Climate Change, Health & Equity (CCHE)	Foundation-funded grant program	15
Kresge Climate Resilient and Equitable Water Systems (CREWS)	Foundation-funded grant program	2
RWJF Global Learning	Foundation-funded grant program	6
RWJF Health and Climate Solutions Program	Foundation-funded grant program	7
Mendez[33]	Journal article	5
National Association of Resilience Planners (NACRP) report[34]	Report	5
California Transformative Climate Communities Program (TCC), UCLA Luskin Center for Innovation	State-funded grant program	4
Public Health Institute (PHI) Stories From the Field	State-funded Web site	2
Other	Web search of California city CAP not funded by state TCC grants	2
Total		48

Note. CAP = Climate Action Plan; RWJF = Robert Wood Johnson Foundation.

version of this article at http://www.ajph.org). Twenty-nine of the CBCAs were led by nonprofit, community-based organizations (CBOs). Eleven of these CBO-led initiatives were formal coalitions of CBOs. Another 6 CBCAs brought together coalitions of CBOs and local government agencies. Local government agencies led 10 CBCAs, 8 of which were city or county agencies; the remaining 2 were led by tribal governments. Entities leading the remaining 3 CBCAs included a community development corporation, a national nonprofit, and a natural history museum.

Focus on Vulnerable and Marginalized Populations

The reports of CBCAs reviewed for this analysis all described working with vulnerable and marginalized populations, an inclusion criterion for our sample. The nature and aims of engaging these groups varied, as did the rationale for focusing on particular populations. Target populations for all CBCAs were reported to have been selected based on their disproportionately high vulnerability, or burden of social, economic, or health disparities. Reviewed reports usually cited characteristics such as low levels of income and high proportion of non-White, typically Black or Latino, residents. Specific social or political marginalization was rarely mentioned as the basis for focusing on a particular group. When marginalization was mentioned as the rationale for focusing on a particular population, such as in accounts of the Oakland [California] Climate Action Coalition and Seattle, Washington's Duwamish Valley Resilience District Project, organizations' efforts overall were framed in terms of broader struggles for social justice and self-determination. Marginalization was also mentioned in Circular Cleveland, a city agency-led initiative in Cleveland, Ohio, aiming to spur economic development with reduced waste and pollution in historically disadvantaged neighborhoods. This was also the only city-led CBCA in the sample that emphasized capacity-building in community engagement efforts.

Engagement of vulnerable groups was usually highly prescribed and tightly circumscribed in CBCAs led by local government agencies. For example, agency-led CBCAs in Austin, Texas, and Albany, New York, reported seeking community input on how public infrastructure and services could better protect residents from floods and heat risks but did not appear to open up dialogue to consider other climate-related risks or resilience-building priorities or strategies for addressing these risks. That said, 1 example of an agency-led CBCA, San Francisco, California's efforts to develop a climate action plan, was both highly prescribed and open to a wide range of input. Another exceptional characteristic of San Francisco's community engagement efforts was their outreach to people with preexisting conditions that would put them at higher risk for climate-related exposures, which was not mentioned in the reports of other CBCAs. Among city-led CBCAs, Seattle's Duwamish Valley Resilience District, which worked with a coalition of community organizations, stood apart for the high level of autonomy given to community members to direct its scope and process.

Building Community Agency

Thirty-three of the 48 CBCAs reported community agency-building activities (Table 2). These were characterized by efforts to enable broader, more effective participation in organizations' climate actions. Epitomizing this approach were descriptions of organizations and communities acting as the subjects rather than the objects of action. An example of this was Green Together's work in Los Angeles, California's Northeast San Fernando Valley to build and strengthen their coalition, providing job training for residents, and conducting train-the-trainer advocacy training.

Aims and context were essential for categorizing community engagement activities. This was sometimes challenging because of our reliance on review of existing reports. One of the clearer examples of capacity-building was the Covenant Pathway Project's efforts to embed climate awareness and adaptation in their community-led regenerative agriculture training for Navajo farmers. Programmatic context is essential for understanding the nature

TABLE 2— Distribution of Health Equity–Focused Community-Based Climate Action (CBCA) Initiatives Categorized by Efforts to Build Community Agency and to Transform Power Relationships, Indicating Type of Health-Equity Focus

Transforming Power Relationships	Building Agency, Focus (No.)		Total No.
	None or Minimal	Yes	
Yes	Inclusion (7)	Transformative Action (12)	19
In flux		Evolving (3)	3
None/minimal	Quasi-Participation (8)	Capacity-Building (18)	26
Total	15	33	48

AJPH February 2023, Vol 113, No. 2

of community engagement activities. A key feature of this project was that it was framed as an effort to develop participants' sense of agency in response to historical oppression.

Transforming Power Relationships

The second dimension of community engagement, transforming power relationships, demonstrated by 19 of the CBCAs (Table 2), was characterized by efforts to increase the power of organizations and the communities that they represented in policy decisions. These ranged from activities aimed at increasing community voice in decision-making, such as get-out-the-vote campaigns and getting community members appointed to local government advisory boards, to efforts to refashion the structure of local government with broader, more inclusive community–agency power-sharing arrangements. As seen in Oakland, the highest levels on this axis are exemplified by a combination of efforts to organize grassroots coalitions (building power from below) and protests at city meetings (dismantling disempowering rules from above). Approaches to transform power were observed in conjunction with efforts to build community agency in 12 of these 19 CBCAs, resulting in the classification of these CBCAs in the Transformative Action quadrant of our typology.

Efforts to transform power combined with vigorous efforts to build agency in the community were broader and more structural in nature. An example of combined agency-building and power transformation, classified as Transformative Action in our typology, was the Oakland Climate Action Coalition's efforts to increase the representation of historically marginalized groups in the city's climate policy decisions. Rather than just seeking inclusion of more community members on city advisory committees, the coalition worked to get city agencies to agree to a model of shared decision-making in which community committees had real decision-making authority, which also involved dismantling existing power structures that excluded community voice and decision-making authority. Furthermore, the coalition worked to increase the breadth and sustainability of this transformation in power relationships by conducing ongoing training workshops for community members to build their knowledge and skills for more effectively participating in this power-sharing.

Without complementary efforts to build capacity and agency, attempts to transform power relationships tended to be narrower in scope. Activities classified as inclusion, marked by efforts to transform power relationships with little or no building of community agency, were exemplified by campaigns, such as the one pursued by Friends of Trees, to get community representatives appointed to advisory boards. Voter education and get-out-the-vote campaigns were similarly categorized as Inclusion. Increasing community voice and representation is a common theme in this category.

Evolving Approaches

Three CBCAs were difficult to categorize into the typology because their efforts were evolving. These 3 CBCAs—Seattle's Duwamish Valley Resilience Project, the Communities of Color Coalition in Portland, Oregon, and the GAVA project in Austin, Texas—were all currently focused primarily on building community agency and capacity, while coupling these efforts with some limited advocacy work. All three framed these efforts as part of an intentional community transformation process, eventually leading to broad community empowerment for climate action. If their efforts were categorized solely on the basis of what was already being done, these CBCAs would best be described as Capacity-Building, but seen in terms of an unfolding process that these groups articulated, this characterization does not fully describe their efforts.

The Duwamish Valley Resilience Project was particularly difficult to categorize. The project aims to introduce a model of shared governance, combining top-down expertise from the city and bottom-up organizing of community groups to improve climate resilience, remediate pollution, and reduce health disparities. Reflecting the necessarily broad scope of climate resilience efforts, the multifaceted, evolving approach of this project seemed particularly open to addressing a broad range of community priorities.

Quasi-Participation

Eight of the CBCAs were classified as Quasi-Participation, based on their lack of reported efforts to build community agency or to transform community power relationships. Half of these CBCAs were led by local government agencies, compared with about one fifth of CBCAs (10 of 48) in the overall sample. They also tended to be very broad in their geographic scope—for example, the City of Los Angeles's efforts to develop a climate action plan and the Regeneration Midwest project that covered 6 states. Compared with other CBCAs, the scope of these CBCAs tended to be sharply defined at the outset, usually narrowly, such as the Alaska Native

Tribal Health Consortium's efforts to install climate-resilient water and sanitation systems and Regeneration Midwest's focus on promoting regenerative farming. These CBCAs were also characterized by a reliance on technical experts and a utilitarian focus on outcomes more than rights and process, as exemplified by the Resilient Corridors project in Lawrence, Massachusetts.

DISCUSSION

Health equity needs to be a central consideration in efforts to limit the human health consequences of climate change in order to limit the widening of health disparities, to build adaptive capacity in communities threatened by climate-related disruptions, and to take advantage of emerging opportunities for promoting climate and health cobenefits.

If health equity is defined as a process of increasing community capacity and power to identify and tackle the causes of ill health, not just a state of reduced health disparities, then community engagement is crucial. The CBCAs in this study sample shared stated goals of reducing climate-related health disparities, but they differed widely in the community engagement processes employed to achieve this goal.

Our 2-dimensional typology of community engagement processes for health equity provides a potentially useful way to understand community initiatives in terms of building community capacity and power. This nonrepresentative, purposive sample included many examples of efforts focused on building community agency. Although some CBCAs worked to transform power relationships—specifically, increasing community voice and authority in community climate policymaking—few CBCAs demonstrated the combination of building internal capacity and transforming external power, labeled Transformative Action in this typology.

Our review did not attempt to ascertain the impact of sampled CBCAs on climate adaptation or resilience. Most of these projects are still in their early implementation phases. We do not know their effectiveness in addressing different threats. The hazards they tackle may also evolve over time. In these early phases, projects in the Quasi-Participation quadrant seemed more likely than others to focus on a narrower, well-defined set of hazards, a choice that may be associated with other differences, such as the availability of funding or level of public agency involvement.

Limitations

The chief limitation of this study is its small, purposive sample, which was neither representative nor all-inclusive. Our aim was to identify exemplars of how health equity–promoting efforts are operationalized, not to estimate the relative frequency of different categories of CBCAs. Because we relied on published reports and grant announcements, we may have omitted categories of CBCAs that are not typically represented in these sources, such as small projects funded wholly by agency funds, as well as more radical or controversial initiatives that did not fall within the scope of what most foundations would consider funding. The sampling approach, which focused on identifying actions carried out as part of well-defined projects, may have also biased the distribution of actions represented in the typology, and may have entirely missed some types of organization-building actions that fall outside the scope of well-defined projects. Reliance on project reports may have also underrepresented such organization-building activities that were seen as more procedural.

Reliance on secondary sources may have also limited the findings in other ways. Inferences were made based on review of project and organization Web sites, funders' reports, and news articles, not from direct observation or from objective assessments. Sources may have emphasized noteworthy accomplishments and underreported setbacks and routine organizing activities. We also had little information on the historical context of most CBCAs. Any CBCA may have been part of a larger initiative that employed a mix of approaches.

We also did not review policies or actions at larger regional, state, federal, or international levels. Policies and initiatives at these larger scales play a huge role in focusing attention, establishing rules, and devoting resources to shape health equity. The latitude of potential action, resources, and, ultimately, the success of local health equity efforts are shaped by policies and resource allocations made by higher levels of government. How health equity efforts manifest in those arenas, however, is entirely different from the local, on-the-ground initiatives analyzed here.

Two lines of research could address the limitations of this preliminary research. In-depth case study research employing a more participatory approach to data collection could provide insights into CBCAs' programmatic and historical context. Such research would also help build agency among participating individuals and organizations, and provide them with ownership of the research. For this current preliminary investigation, however, which spanned multiple actions in multiple communities, such a participatory approach would have been logistically challenging. Eventually, large-scale systematic longitudinal sampling of equity-focused community initiatives could also help understand the long-term impacts of the different community, organizational, and individual processes identified in the typology. Researchers and practitioners will also need to examine how community engagement around climate issues might differ from community engagement around other, more localized public health issues. Although local climate actions and impacts are important, the long-term and global context of climate threats and responses adds a layer of complexity to these efforts.

Public Health Implications

The typology of health equity–supporting CBCA focuses attention on processes that advance health equity as part of local climate actions. It can be used to diagnose gaps, plan responses, and track the progress of efforts to improve health equity. Moving beyond rhetoric, this typology suggests concrete steps toward building community agency and power for advancing health equity. Community organizations could use it to plan and prioritize actions, guide process evaluations, and articulate to funders how their proposals will contribute to health equity. Funders could incorporate elements of this typology into requests for proposals, requesting that applicants detail specific actions to build community agency and power that are being proposed and explain how changes in each will be measured.

Although corporate, national, and transnational actions are also needed to address the climate crisis, robust community engagement cannot be neglected in efforts to advance health equity and to enable vulnerable and marginalized communities to confront the challenges of climate change. AJPH

ABOUT THE AUTHORS

Brian L. Cole is with the Health Science Department, California State University, Long Beach, and the Center for Healthy Climate Solutions, University of California, Los Angeles. Irish Del Rosario is with the Department of Epidemiology, Fielding School of Public Health, University of California, Los Angeles. Astrid Hendricks is with BCT Partners, Pasadena, CA. David P. Eisenman is with the Division of General Internal Medicine and Health Services Research, David Geffen School of Medicine, and the Centers for Public Health and Disasters and Healthy Climate Solutions, Fielding School of Public Health, University of California, Los Angeles.

CORRESPONDENCE

Correspondence should be sent to Brian L. Cole, Health Science Department, California State University, Long Beach, 1250 Bellflower Blvd, Long Beach, CA 90840 (e-mail: brian.cole@csulb.edu). Reprints can be ordered at http://www.ajph.org by clicking the "Reprints" link.

PUBLICATION INFORMATION

Full Citation: Cole BL, Del Rosario I, Hendricks A, Eisenman DP. Advancing health equity in community-based climate action: from concept to practice. *Am J Public Health*. 2023;113(2): 185–193.

Acceptance Date: October 2, 2022.

DOI: https://doi.org/10.2105/AJPH.2022.307143

CONTRIBUTORS

All authors jointly conceptualized the study and reviewed and edited the article. B. L. Cole drafted most sections of the article and developed the typology. I. Del Rosario led the assembly and analysis of data on the cases with assistance from B. L. Cole and A. Hendricks. D. P. Eisenman worked with B. L. Cole to draft the Discussion section.

ACKNOWLEDGMENTS

The Robert Wood Johnson Foundation Health and Climate Solutions Program provided funding for this study.

CONFLICTS OF INTEREST

The authors have no financial or other conflicts of interest to disclose.

HUMAN PARTICIPANT PROTECTION

This study reviewed publicly available organization reports and did not involve any human participant research.

REFERENCES

1. Atwoli L, Baqui AH, Benfield T, et al. Call for emergency action to limit global temperature increases, restore biodiversity, and protect health. *BMJ Glob Health*. 2021;6(9):e007228. https://doi.org/10.1136/bmjgh-2021-007228
2. Costello A, Abbas M, Allen A, et al. Managing the health effects of climate change: Lancet and University College London Institute for Global Health Commission. *Lancet*. 2009;373(9676):1693–1733. https://doi.org/10.1016/S0140-6736(09)60935-1
3. Füssel HM. How inequitable is the global distribution of responsibility, capability, and vulnerability to climate change: a comprehensive indicator-based assessment. *Glob Environ Change*. 2010;20(4): 597–611. https://doi.org/10.1016/j.gloenvcha.2010.07.009
4. Bikomeye JC, Rublee CS, Beyer KMM. Positive externalities of climate change mitigation and adaptation for human health: a review and conceptual framework for public health research. *Int J Environ Res Public Health*. 2021;18(5):2481. https://doi.org/10.3390/ijerph18052481
5. Patz JA, Gibbs HK, Foley JA, Rogers JV, Smith KR. Climate change and global health: quantifying a growing ethical crisis. *EcoHealth*. 2007;4(4):397–405. https://doi.org/10.1007/s10393-007-0141-1
6. US Environmental Protection Agency. Climate change and social vulnerability in the United States: a focus on six impacts. 2021. Available at: https://www.epa.gov/system/files/documents/2021-09/climate-vulnerability_september-2021_508.pdf. Accessed January 26, 2022.
7. Pelling M, Chow WTL, Chu E, et al. A climate resilience research renewal agenda: learning lessons from the COVID-19 pandemic for urban climate resilience. *Clim Dev*. 2021;14(7):1–8. https://doi.org/10.1080/17565529.2021.1956411
8. Haines A. Health co-benefits of climate action. *Lancet Planet Health*. 2017;1(1):e4–e5. https://doi.org/10.1016/S2542-5196(17)30003-7
9. Scovronick N, Budolfson M, Dennig F, et al. The impact of human health co-benefits on evaluations of global climate policy. *Nat Commun*. 2019; 10(1):1095. https://doi.org/10.1038/s41467-019-09499-x
10. Liburd LC, Hall JE, Mpofu JJ, Williams SM, Bouye K, Penman-Aguilar A. Addressing health equity in public health practice: frameworks, promising strategies, and measurement considerations. *Annu Rev Public Health*. 2020;41(1):417–432. https://doi.org/10.1146/annurev-publhealth-040119-094119
11. Braveman P. What are health disparities and health equity? We need to be clear. *Public Health Rep*. 2014;129(suppl 2):5–8. https://doi.org/10.1177/00333549141291S203
12. Angelo H, Macfarlane K, Sirigotis J. *The Challenge of Equity in California's Municipal Climate Action Plans Resilient Optionality: (Infra)Structures of Water*. Santa Cruz: University of California, Santa Cruz, Institute for Social Transformation; 2020. https://doi.org/10.13140/RG.2.2.33886.25920

13. Braveman P, Arkin E, Orleans T, Proctor D, Plough A. What is health equity? And what difference does a definition make? Robert Wood Johnson Foundation. 2017. Available at: https://www.rwjf.org/en/library/research/2017/05/what-is-health-equity-.html. Accessed January 26, 2022.
14. Moser SC, Pike C. Community engagement on adaptation: meeting a growing capacity need. *Urban Clim.* 2015;14:111–115. https://doi.org/10.1016/j.uclim.2015.06.006
15. Rouse HL, Bell RG, Lundquist CJ, Blackett PE, Hicks DM, King DN. Coastal adaptation to climate change in Aotearoa-New Zealand. *N Z J Marine Freshwater Res.* 2017;51(2):183–222. https://doi.org/10.1080/00288330.2016.1185736
16. *Closing the Gap in a Generation: Health Equity Through Action on the Social Determinants of Health. Final Report of the Commission on Social Determinants of Health.* Geneva, Switzerland: World Health Organization; 2008.
17. Rifkin SB. A framework linking community empowerment and health equity: it is a matter of CHOICE. *J Health Popul Nutr.* 2003;21(3):168–180. http://www.jstor.org/stable/23499215
18. Sardenberg CMB. Liberal vs liberating empowerment: a Latin American feminist perspective on conceptualising women's empowerment. *IDS Bull.* 2008;39(6):18–27. https://doi.org/10.1111/j.1759-5436.2008.tb00507.x
19. Partzsch L. "Power with" and "power to" in environmental politics and the transition to sustainability. *Env Polit.* 2017;26(2):193–211. https://doi.org/10.1080/09644016.2016.1256961
20. Bradley A. Did we forget about power? Reintroducing concepts of power for justice, equality and peace. In: McGee R, Pettit J, eds. *Power, Empowerment and Social Change.* New York, NY: Routledge; 2019:101–116. https://doi.org/10.4324/9781351272322-7
21. Gaventa J. Linking the prepositions: using power analysis to inform strategies for social action. *J Polit Power.* 2021;14(1):109–130. https://doi.org/10.1080/2158379X.2021.1878409
22. Arnstein SR. A ladder of citizen participation. *J Am Plann Assoc.* 1969;35(4):216–224. https://doi.org/10.1080/01944366908977225
23. Pateman C. *Participation and Democratic Theory.* Cambridge, UK: Cambridge University Press; 1970. https://doi.org/10.1017/CBO9780511720444
24. Tritter JQ, McCallum A. The snakes and ladders of user involvement: moving beyond Arnstein. *Health Policy.* 2006;76(2):156–168. https://doi.org/10.1016/j.healthpol.2005.05.008
25. Rothman J. Multi modes of intervention at the macro level. *J Community Pract.* 2007;15(4):11–40. https://doi.org/10.1300/J125v15n04_02
26. Minkler M, Wallerstein N, Wilson N. Community organizing and community building for health and welfare. In: Minkler M, ed. *Community Organizing and Community Building for Health and Welfare.* 3rd ed. New Brunswick, NJ: Rutgers University Press; 2012:287–312. https://doi.org/10.36019/9780813553146
27. Walter CL, Hyde CA. Community building practice: an expanded conceptual framework. In: Minkler M, ed. *Community Organizing and Community Building for Health and Welfare.* 3rd ed. New Brunswick, NJ: Rutgers University Press; 2012:78–90.
28. Newman L, Dale A. The role of agency in sustainable local community development. *Local Environ.* 2005;10(5):477–486. https://doi.org/10.1080/13549830500203121
29. Lukes S. *Power: A Radical View.* 2nd ed. Basingstoke, UK: Macmillan; 2005.
30. Cornwall A, Edwards J. Introduction: negotiating Empowerment. *IDS Bull.* 2010;41(2):1–9. https://doi.org/10.1111/j.1759-5436.2010.00117.x
31. Stockdale JD. Community organization practice: an elaboration of Rothman's typology. *J Sociol Soc Welf.* 1975;3:541–555.
32. Morgan MA, Lifshay J. Community engagement in public health. Available at: https://cchealth.org/public-health/pdf/community_engagement_in_ph.pdf. Accessed August 7, 2022.
33. Mendez MA. Assessing local climate action plans for public health co-benefits in environmental justice communities. *Local Environ.* 2015;20(6):637–663. https://doi.org/10.1080/13549839.2015.1038227
34. Gonzalez R, James T, Ross J. Community-driven climate resilience planning: a framework. Version 2.0. 2017. Available at: http://www.nacrp.org. Accessed March 1, 2022.

Health Justice: A Framework for Mitigating the Impacts of HIV and COVID-19 on Disproportionately Affected Communities

Sirry Alang, PhD, and Oni Blackstock, MD, MHS

See also Fereidooni et al., p. 228, Ferreira and Buttell, p. 136, and Kapadia, p. 144.

Health crises have a disproportionate impact on communities that are marginalized by systems of oppression such as racism and capitalism. Benefits of advances such as in the prevention and treatment of HIV disease are unequally distributed. Intersecting factors including poverty, homophobia, homelessness, racism, and mass incarceration expose marginalized populations to greater risks while limiting access to resources that buffer these risks. Similar patterns have emerged with COVID-19.

We identify comparable pitfalls in our responses to HIV and COVID-19. We introduce health justice as a framework for mitigating the long-term impact of the HIV epidemic and COVID-19 pandemic. The health justice framework considers the central role of power in the health and liberation of communities hit hardest by legacies of marginalization.

We provide 5 recommendations grounded in health justice: (1) redistribute resources, (2) enforce mandates that redistribute power, (3) enact legislation that guarantees support for people with long-haul COVID-19, (4) center experiences of the most impacted communities in policy development, and (5) evaluate multidimensional effects of policies across systems. Successful implementation of these recommendations requires community organizing and collective action. (*Am J Public Health*. 2023;113(2): 194–201. https://doi.org/10.2105/AJPH.2022.307139)

AJPH February 2023, Vol 113, No. 2

Communities marginalized by structural inequities often experience a disproportionate burden of disease. This is true for HIV and for COVID-19. About 1.2 million people are living with HIV in the United States, with almost 35 000 new infections each year.[1] In 2019, Black Americans accounted for 44% of new HIV diagnoses, although they comprise 13% of the US population. Latino/a/x Americans make up 18% of the population but account for 30% of new cases.[1] Rates of HIV infection are high in communities harmed by structural racism and other forms of oppression.[2–4] Evidence from a systematic review of studies worldwide suggests that people living with HIV have an elevated risk of contracting severe acute respiratory syndrome coronavirus 2 (SARS-CoV-2), the cause of COVID-19, and that they have a higher risk of COVID-19 mortality compared with persons who are not HIV-positive.[5]

HIV and COVID-19 coinfection is likely to increase, and communities hit hardest by systemic oppression such as poverty, racism, homophobia, transphobia, misogyny, homelessness, addiction, residential segregation, food insecurity, mass incarceration, and so forth will continue to bear most of the burden of these public health crises.[3,4] Here, we identify comparable pitfalls in responses to HIV and COVID-19 in the United States. We also offer the health justice framework as the central component of our recommended strategies for mitigating the long-term impact of the burdens of the HIV epidemic and COVID-19 pandemic on communities marginalized by structural inequities.

DIFFERENT VIRUSES, SIMILAR RESPONSE PITFALLS

Strategies employed to address COVID-19 are not new. In a lot of ways, these strategies are leading to similar outcomes that emerged from our national response to HIV.

Initial Nonresponse

Following the first confirmed case of COVID-19 in the United States, the Centers for Disease Control and Prevention (CDC) stated that they have "been proactively preparing for the introduction of 2019-nCoV in the United States."[6] This press release was different from CDC's first publication about HIV in that there was no preparation for what later developed into an epidemic. Reporting the presence of a rare cancer and a rare pneumonia-like disease that killed young gay men, the CDC hypothesized that the virus was contained in seminal fluid and that the disease occurred predominantly among gay men.[7]

The initial national response was a nonresponse reflecting attitudes about those who were being disproportionately affected—gay men. Writing about how this nonresponse led to a global humanitarian crisis, Greg Behrman, a former US State Department official, stated:

> The subpopulations suffering in the United States were not part of Reagan's constituency. . . . If the disease was truly heterosexual, then it was a bigger problem (at least politically) than the administration had estimated. They would have to address it, and they didn't want to do that unless they had to.[8(p27)]

It was not until 4 years after the crisis began that President Reagan finally acknowledged AIDS in public.[8]

President Trump's initial nonresponse to COVID-19 had a similar effect. On January 22, 2020, 2 days after the CDC confirmed the first case in the United States, President Trump stated: "We have it totally under control. It's one person coming in from China. It's going to be just fine."[9] A month later, at different occasions, he stated: "Coronavirus is very much under control in the USA . . . the Stock Market starting to look very good to me!" "I think that's a problem that's going to go away. . . . They have studied it. They know very much. In fact, we're very close to a vaccine." "The 15 [cases in the United States] within a couple of days is going to be down to close to zero."[9] President Trump's underestimation of the virus was different from President Reagan's dissociation from HIV, which was fueled by widespread homophobia and moral panic around gay male sexuality. However, both presidents were motivated by what was best for them politically, not what was best for public health. Their nonresponses meant no federal public health action, thereby exacerbating suffering.

Structural Determinants of Risk Factors Ignored

Public discussions, medical recommendations, and political actions around HIV did not initially consider the structural drivers of HIV vulnerability. For example, lack of structural and material support such as housing, the absence of social support, employment and housing discrimination, and the criminalization of homosexuality, sex work, and substance use all increase the risk of contracting HIV but were not emphasized.[10] The focus was predominantly on the social identities of people who were infected. Indeed, at the beginning of the epidemic, the CDC referred to groups being impacted by HIV as the "Four Hs"—"homosexuals, heroin users, hemophiliacs, and Haitians."[11] However, understanding how structural inequities shape the actions of people with specific social identities and increase exposure to risk is critical. Unfortunately, most of the early epidemiological literature on HIV centered on these groups, sending a message that only people with specific identities were vulnerable. Identities, not structural factors, were highlighted as risk factors. HIV was not an "everyone's disease."

With COVID-19, early messaging was that it was indeed everyone's disease—that we were all in this together. But epidemics highlight and exacerbate existing structural inequities.[3,12] As more data became available, it was evident that Black, Latino/a/x, and Indigenous communities; persons living in poverty; people in predominantly underresourced neighborhoods; and those working in the health care sector or who lived with essential workers were disproportionately more likely to be infected, to be hospitalized, and to die from COVID-19.[3,13] Structural racism—how our institutions, culture, ideology, norms, and practices create and maintain racial dominance and oppression through the control of resources, producing adverse and racially inequitable outcomes—drives the unjust burden of COVID-19 on racially minoritized groups.[3,4,14] And capital accumulation limits access to resources needed to work from home and afford high-quality masks and regular at-home tests.[3,14] These larger systemic factors drive inequities in COVID-19 outcomes. However, our national response focuses heavily on individual behaviors.

Blaming Victims

Significant blame has been assigned to groups who contract HIV for whom there is some level of societal moral disapproval of their behaviors. Examples include men who have sex with men, sex workers, and injection drug users. Similarly, people who have not received COVID-19 vaccines and those who have no choice but to continue to go to work when exposed or sick are usually perceived as responsible for why things are not "back to normal." Underrepresentation of the working class in political processes and resistance to policies such as Medicare for All that are likely to facilitate engagement in healthy behaviors and access to care also increase the tendency to see risks as products of individual choices rather than outcomes of the political contexts.

The ability of the most privileged and insulated members of society to work from home or stay at home when exposed, for example, is attributable to less-privileged members assuming more risks because of the absence of social policies and safety-net programs that protect them.[15] Attributing a public health crisis to individual actions distracts from the structural issues that matter more,[16,17] causing our policy responses to unfortunately center individual responsibility even when personal agency is significantly constrained by structural factors. Blaming individual actions that are risky such as going to social gatherings is both politically convenient and driven by capitalism. For example, government avoids imposing restrictions on big businesses and employers. Victim blaming might also contribute to fear and reluctance to seek care, leading to further suffering.

Profits Over People

One of the most devasting things about the HIV epidemic is that it could have been stopped sooner by making lifesaving antiretroviral therapy (ART) accessible to sub-Saharan Africa, Central and South America, and India, where HIV prevalence rates were highest.[8] Driven by capitalism, pharmaceutical companies in wealthy countries colluded with international organizations such as the World Trade Organization and with some leaders of Western countries to set policies around manufacturing and distribution of ART that kept these medications out of the reach of people who needed them the most. Access to ART motivates people to get tested, decreases rates of transmission by reducing viral load, and prevents progression to AIDS.[18] It was only until after years of HIV activism that generic drugs were finally allowed to be imported by countries without previous access to medications.[8] By then, it was too late for many. The toll was already devastating.

The lack of global access to COVID-19 vaccines mirrors the lack of global access to ART for HIV. When vaccines first became available, several groups warned that these vaccines would not be available to people living in impoverished countries as pharmaceutical companies would not share the formula so that they could maximize profits as wealthy countries hoarded vaccines. Indeed, wealthy countries were negotiating advance purchasing deals before the vaccines were even approved.[19] Stockpiling of vaccine doses by wealthy countries while many in poorer countries remain unvaccinated increases odds of additional variants of concern.

Inequities in access to HIV treatment (ART), preexposure prophylaxis (PrEP), and COVID-19 vaccines are also prevalent in the United States. For example, Black and Latino men who have sex with men have less access to PrEP and ART than their White peers.[2,20] And economically marginalized populations have lower COVID-19 vaccination rates compared with high-income populations.[21] Nothing indicates our prioritization of profits over people more than the fact that one's ability to access lifesaving medications and vaccinations depends on access to money, the politics of where they live, and other flexible resources.

THE HEALTH JUSTICE FRAMEWORK

We propose the health justice framework as the basis for sustainable, equitable, and ethical responses to HIV and COVID-19. Drawing from intersectionality theory,[22–24] the framework is premised on the assumption that all systems (e.g., capitalism, racism, homophobia, misogyny, xenophobia), all structures (e.g., race, gender, class, sexuality), and all institutions (e.g., political, economic, social) matter for health and well-being. As shown in Figure 1, these structures, systems, and institutions intersect to create and maintain unequal distribution of power and access to and distribution of resources that matter for health.

We conceptualize health justice as the equitable redistribution of power and resources such that people with the greatest need are prioritized, and where the processes of knowledge production around need, restructuring, and redistribution are grounded in the experiences of populations most impacted by health inequities. Health justice is a paradigm and collection of actions that interrogate systems; structures; social, political, economic, and cultural institutions; and networks of relationships that, although normalized, create and perpetuate inequities in power and access to resources that matter for health, including the ability to engage in healthy behaviors.

It is different from health equity in that it extends beyond removing obstacles and beyond giving everyone a fair

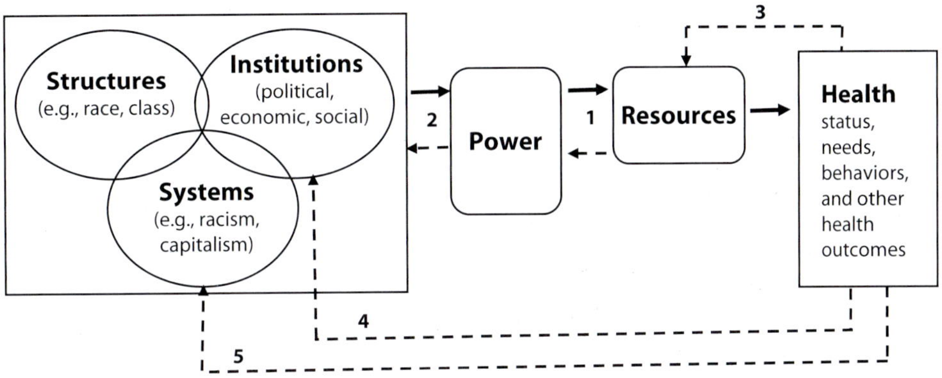

1. Redistribute resources to ensure that health needs of people who are negatively impacted by oppressive systems are met.
2. Redistribute power to increase access to resources *and* to disrupt systems, structures, and institutions that cause the unequal distribution of power.
3. Enact legislation that guarantees support for people with long-haul COVID-19 to ensure that they have access to material, social, and structural resources that matter for their health and sustenance in the long term.
4. Center the experiences of the most impacted communities—communities with the worst outcomes—to ensure that they have power, that they influence the development of institutional policies, *and* that these policies will meet their needs.
5. Evaluate intersecting and multidimensional effects of policies across systems to make sure new inequities and new mechanisms of oppression are not produced.

FIGURE 1— Policy Recommendations Based on the Health Justice Framework

opportunity to be healthy.[25] It is also distinct from previous conceptualizations of health justice that focus on recognizing the human and civil rights of everyone.[25] Specifically, our conceptualization of health justice considers how barriers to health occur because people with more power (ability to control resources and shape how the society is structured, whether that power is conferred by statuses such as occupation or by structures such as race) and access to resources (e.g., social, economic, material, political) benefit at the expense of people with less power and resources.

Addressing barriers to well-being from a health justice perspective requires people and institutions with the most power to reject the benefits of their power and to work toward relinquishing that power altogether—a feature that distinguishes health justice from health equity and health as a human right. For example, the ability of multibillion-dollar corporations to amass wealth during a pandemic comes at the expense of workers who have no choice but to return to work after a positive coronavirus test. The ability to get groceries delivered comes at a cost to essential workers and low-income factory workers. While one's job might be because they attended a good school or because someone "put in a good word" for them, it all comes at the expense of someone else who might be just as smart and hardworking, but who could not attend a resource-rich school because of structural factors like residential segregation or the lack of networks that facilitate desirable employment. The health justice framework certainly complicates the idea that none of us is free until all of us are free. While we agree that interconnectedness of systems and institutions means that we are deeply implicated in each other's lives, we also argue that some of us are only free because some of us are oppressed. Therefore, the health justice framework seeks liberation, restitution, and advancement for communities hit hardest by legacies of marginalization.

STRATEGIES FOR THE PATH FORWARD

Public health policies are more effective when implemented by federal, state, and local levels of government.[26] While we identify 5 policy recommendations to help eliminate health inequities caused by HIV and COVID-19, we concede that political forces in the United States (e.g., filibuster, gerrymandering, and corporate lobbying) are significant obstacles to implementing these. Community organizing and collaborations between public–private and nonprofit sectors are important for public health[27–29]; hence, they are necessary for the implementation of the recommendations we propose in Figure 1.

Redistribution of Resources

People who are disproportionately affected by HIV and COVID-19 are often marginalized and oppressed. Hence, they do not have resources to effect their own liberation. This is where government should come in. The United States is taking an approach to ending the pandemic that still largely relies on individual choices and resources. In March of 2022, the White House released the National COVID-19 Preparedness Plan,[30] an updated plan to meet current challenges. The first goal of the revised plan was to protect against and treat COVID-19 by encouraging testing, wearing masks when risks of transmission are high, and increasing access to vaccines, high-quality masks, and lifesaving antiviral pills. To a large degree, frequent testing, wearing masks, and getting vaccinated are contingent upon personal resources and preferences.

One major failure in our response to the HIV epidemic is we only focused on behavioral changes while not providing resources such as universal health care and needle-exchange programs that make behavioral modifications possible and sustainable.[3,8] Fortunately, rapid tests for COVID-19, vaccines, and high-filtration masks have become more available. However, accessing them still relies on individual resources. For example, people who are insured have relatively easier access to free tests compared with those who are uninsured. Similarly, ordering and receiving free test kits from the government requires access to the Internet and a home address. COVID-19 is transmitted by an airborne virus. Thus, the quality of ventilation in buildings such as schools and offices matters. The likelihood of working from home or in buildings with good air circulation is partially dependent on one's socioeconomic status.

We call on the Biden administration to expand the distribution of high-quality masks, tests, vaccines, and medications, especially for populations in low-wage, high-risk essential jobs. Legacies of marginalization ensure that people most at risk also have limited resources including specialized knowledge and time to find the free home test kits, masks, and medications that are available. Government has a responsibility to provide resources, to develop infrastructure and strategies that will connect these resources to people who need them the most, and to mandate employers to do the same. Resources to improve ventilation and air filtration in buildings, including access to portable air cleaners, should be made available.

Redistribute Power

We must truly prioritize people over profits. One of the goals of the COVID-19 Preparedness Plan is to prevent economic and educational shutdowns by keeping schools and businesses safely open.[30] Two months before the release of the revised preparedness plan, the CDC shortened the isolation period from 10 days to 5 days for those who test positive for SARS-CoV-2. However, the ways by which prioritization of the economy undermine collective health and well-being and increase the risk of community transmission are not considered. One of the 10 essential public health services is to utilize legal and regulatory actions to improve and protect the health of the public.[31] The government has power to enforce regulations for schools and multibillion-dollar industries alike. People most negatively impacted do not have the power to restructure institutions and policies in ways that would facilitate their liberation. This requires the Biden administration to develop and enforce regulations to protect health.

Government has a history of regulating all kinds of activities when politically convenient. Driven by homophobia and the need to control the sexuality of gay men, bathhouses and gay bars were shut down, and gay men were banned from donating blood as the government argued that these were critical in curbing the spread of HIV.[32] Currently, there are no mandates or enforceable policies that regulate congregation of people indoors or on airplanes. Masks are optional. Masking when indoors or when in crowds is an individual choice shaped by politics.[33] And people who might be unvaccinated, immunocompromised, or otherwise more susceptible to the virus are still at greater risks and remain unprotected.

We recommend workplace safety standards, mask mandates and capacity limits for indoor public gatherings, vaccine mandates for domestic flights, and paid time off for up to 10 days for people who have tested positive for SARS-CoV-2, pay that is supplemented by the federal government and from a proportion of profits and net revenues of large, wealthy employers.

Enact Legislation for People With Long-Haul COVID-19

Significant funds should be made available to specifically support the growing number of people who are unable to work because of long COVID-19–related limitations. One of the most significant national policy responses to HIV was the enactment of the Ryan White Program, which pays for medical and support services for low-income persons living with HIV. A similar legislation should be enacted for long-term medical and support services that are needed by people who are navigating COVID-19–related disabilities, unable to work, or in precarious employment situations with no benefits to support comprehensive rehabilitation services.

At the state level, Medicaid expansion is also necessary, especially as it is likely to cover a more comprehensive set of services for those who, because of the undue burden of COVID-19, have become eligible for Medicaid. Southern states that have not expanded Medicaid are also states with relatively high HIV prevalence and greater incidence of COVID-19.[4] Ultimately, universal health care, Medicare for all, or some version of a single-payer system is needed. It is time to restructure our health care system such that access to health services for most persons in the United States is not contingent upon resources such as employment.

Center Most-Impacted Communities

We must center disproportionately affected communities in policy development and implementation. One successful response to HIV is that people living with HIV are involved in informing, developing, implementing, and monitoring programs and policies.[4] For example, for organizations to obtain Part A funds from the Ryan White Program (funds that support HIV services in urban areas), there are requirements for these organizations to demonstrate mechanisms through which people living with HIV participate in needs assessment, prioritization of services, and allocation of funds to these services. A similar requirement that policy and program responses to COVID-19 should have a process for community leadership in planning, implementation, and monitoring is necessary. The experiences of patients with long-haul COVID-19 and their advocates will play a central role in ensuring people with long COVID-19 are supported.[34]

Evaluate Policies Across Systems

We must consider how benefits of our responses to COVID-19 might be inequitably distributed, thus exacerbating other inequities. With HIV, for example, the development of ART and PrEP increased viral suppression and reduced new infections in general but widened racial inequities in viral suppression rates and rates of new infections because, compared with Black and Latino men who have sex with men, White men who have sex with men had more access to these medications.[2,3,20] When there is a new development that prevents disease and death, people with more resources are usually those who can take advantage of these developments. They benefit the most because resources, whether social, financial, or technological, are usually transferable and can be used in many different situations to ultimately improve health.[14]

Access to vaccines, high-filtration masks, and test kits by people with resources can widen existing inequities in COVID-19 outcomes. They can also widen socioeconomic inequities as persons with access to vaccines, masks, and tests likely have greater odds of staying healthy, continuing to work, attending classes, and so forth. Similarly, increase in the use of telemedicine and the move to virtual work and school might create new inequities in learning outcomes and health care utilization. While these developments and measures are critical for controlling the pandemic, we need monitoring systems in place to understand, mitigate, and eliminate new inequities.

CONCLUSION

The health justice framework considers the central role of power and resources in the liberation and advancement of communities who are disproportionately affected by health crises, including those caused by noncommunicable diseases and other conditions—power to make decisions that can affect a broad range of systems, institutions, structures, and populations. Power to make decisions and to control resources needed to support these decisions can alter the trajectories of crises. Government has power to enact far-reaching regulations and mandates and to develop and enforce policies. Government can also make resources available and accessible by regulating and taxing large corporations; by providing supplements, subsidies, and tax reliefs to individuals and businesses; and through the enactment of policies and programs that enable people to save money.

Both HIV and COVID-19 have wrought significant loss, grief, trauma, and suffering. Communities hit hardest by legacies of marginalization are disproportionately affected and should lead the development of long-term solutions. Investing in community-based participatory research now is essential so that communities can begin to direct and work with researchers to identify and prioritize their needs, to develop context-specific approaches to address these needs, and to work toward liberation and advancement. In 40 years, we have made significant advances in HIV prevention and treatment. Yet, the benefits of these advances are not equally distributed. We are seeing the same patterns with COVID-19 in which the benefits of advances such as vaccines, at-home test kits, and medications are unequally distributed. This is compounded by the fact that communities already disproportionately burdened by the HIV pandemic are also burdened by COVID-19.

We need an equitable society to prevent disproportionate impact of health crises. The Coronavirus Tax Relief in the form of economic impact payments and the advance child tax credits helped restore some of the income losses incurred by individuals and families. However, broad structural changes are necessary for the liberation of marginalized populations and for significant long-term benefits that can finally end legacies of marginalization. This is an issue of justice. This is also within our reach. People, systems, and institutions that benefit from structural inequalities at the expense of marginalized communities have a responsibility to relinquish these benefits to level the socioeconomic field.

In the end, government has the utmost responsibility to act decisively by investing in policies that address multiple dimensions of inequality. Policies such as universal health care, guaranteed living wage, universal access to broadband Internet, universal access to childcare regardless of employment status and income, and guaranteed and expanded sick leave will go a long way toward achieving a more equitable society. But government will not act simply because we wish for action. Community organizing; building grassroots movements; advocacy; public, private, and nonprofit collaborations; and grassroots activism are necessary strategies to influence change, even at different levels of government.[16,35,36]

The abolition movement, for example, has been successful in bringing the idea of abolition into the mainstream. People are actively talking about police and prison abolition, and we have seen a few jurisdictions redistribute funding away from policing.[37] Similarly, collective power and action have led to changes in local, state, and federal-level policies that have improved, even incrementally, the health of many constituents such as nonsmokers, persons with disabilities, and people living with HIV.[38] Amid political resistance to change and in the absence of governmental action, movement building and community organizing are critical. AJPH

ABOUT THE AUTHORS

Sirry Alang is with the Department of Health and Human Development at the University of Pittsburgh, Pittsburgh, PA. Oni Blackstock is with Health Justice, New York, NY.

CORRESPONDENCE

Correspondence should be sent to Sirry Alang, PhD, Department of Health and Human Development, University of Pittsburgh School of Education, 5100 Wesley W. Posvar Hall, 230 S Bouquet St, Pittsburgh, PA 15260 (e-mail: salang@pitt.edu). Reprints can be ordered at https://ajph.org by clicking the "Reprints" link.

PUBLICATION INFORMATION

Full Citation: Alang S, Blackstock O. Health justice: a framework for mitigating the impacts of HIV and COVID-19 on disproportionately affected communities. *Am J Public Health*. 2023;113(2):194–201.

Acceptance Date: September 26, 2022.

DOI: https://doi.org/10.2105/AJPH.2022.307139

CONTRIBUTORS

S. Alang conceptualized the article. S. Alang and O. Blackstock contributed equally to writing and editing the article.

ACKNOWLEDGMENTS

The authors thank Lisa Bowleg, PhD, for the extensive and helpful comments on the first version of this article.

CONFLICTS OF INTEREST

There are no conflicts of interest.

HUMAN PARTICIPANT PROTECTION

Human participants were not involved.

REFERENCES

1. Centers for Disease Control and Prevention. HIV surveillance report, 2019. 2021. Available at: http://www.cdc.gov/hiv/library/reports/hiv-surveillance.html. Accessed February 21, 2022.
2. Doshi RK, Bowleg L, Blankenship KM. Tying structural racism to human immunodeficiency virus viral suppression. *Clin Infect Dis*. 2021;72(10):e646–e648. https://doi.org/10.1093/cid/ciaa1252
3. Spinner GF. The intersection of HIV, COVID-19 and systemic racism. *J Health Dispar Res Pract*. 2021;14(2):8.
4. Blackstock OJ. Ensuring progress toward ending the HIV epidemic while confronting the dual pandemics of COVID-19 and systemic racism. *Am J Public Health*. 2021;111(8):1462–1464. https://doi.org/10.2105/AJPH.2021.306196
5. Ssentongo P, Heilbrunn ES, Ssentongo AE, et al. Epidemiology and outcomes of COVID-19 in HIV-infected individuals: a systematic review and meta-analysis. *Sci Rep*. 2021;11(1):628. https://doi.org/10.1038/s41598-021-85359-3
6. Centers for Disease Control and Prevention. First travel-related case of 2019 novel coronavirus detected in United States. January 21, 2020. Available at: https://www.cdc.gov/media/releases/2020/p0121-novel-coronavirus-travel-case.html. Accessed November 4, 2021.
7. Centers for Disease Control and Prevention. Pneumocystis pneumonia—Los Angeles. *MMWR Morb Mortal Wkly Rep*. 1981;30(21):250–252.
8. Behrman G. *The Invisible People: How the US Has Slept Through the Global AIDS Pandemic, the Greatest Humanitarian Catastrophe of Our Time*. New York, NY: Simon and Schuster; 2008.
9. Gore D, Kiely E, Robertson L, Rieder R. Timeline of Trump's COVID-19 comments. October 2, 2020. FactCheck.org. Available at: https://www.factcheck.org/2020/10/timeline-of-trumps-covid-19-comments. Accessed March 3, 2021.
10. Curran JW, Jaffe HW, Hardy AM, Morgan WM, Selik RM, Dondero TJ. Epidemiology of HIV infection and AIDS in the United States. *Science*. 1988;239(4840):610–616. https://doi.org/10.1126/science.3340847
11. Bazell R. Research rewrites first chapter of AIDS in US. *NBC News*. November 6, 2007. Available at: https://www.nbcnews.com/id/wbna21653369. Accessed March 3, 2021.
12. Bowleg L. We're not all in this together: on COVID-19, intersectionality, and structural inequality. *Am J Public Health*. 2020;110(7):917. https://doi.org/10.2105/AJPH.2020.305766
13. Tan SB, DeSouza P, Raifman M. Structural racism and COVID-19 in the USA: a county-level empirical analysis. *J Racial Ethn Health Disparities*. 2022;9(1):236–246. https://doi.10.1007/s40615-020-00948-8
14. Laster Pirtle WN. Racial capitalism: a fundamental cause of novel coronavirus (COVID-19) pandemic inequities in the United States. *Health Educ Behav*. 2020;47(4):504–508. https://doi.org/10.1177/1090198120922942
15. Navarro V. What is happening in the United States? How social classes influence the political

life of the country and its health and quality of life. *Int J Health Serv.* 2021;51(2):125–134. https://doi.org/10.1177/0020731421994841

16. Bassett MT. Tired of science being ignored? Get political. *Nature.* 2020;586(7829):337. https://doi.org/10.1038/d41586-020-02854-9
17. Antonio-Villa NE, Fernandez-Chirino L, Pisanty-Alatorre J, et al. Comprehensive evaluation of the impact of sociodemographic inequalities on adverse outcomes and excess mortality during the coronavirus disease 2019 (COVID-19) pandemic in Mexico City. *Clin Infect Dis.* 2022;74(5):785–792. https://doi.org/10.1093/cid/ciab577
18. Nguyen V-K, Bajos N, Dubois-Arber F, O'Malley J, Pirkle CM. Remedicalizing an epidemic: from HIV treatment as prevention to HIV treatment is prevention. *AIDS.* 2011;25(3):291–293. https://doi.org/10.1097/QAD.0b013e3283402c3e
19. Dyer O. COVID-19: many poor countries will see almost no vaccine next year, aid groups warn. *BMJ.* 2020;371:m4809. https://doi.org/10.1136/bmj.m4809
20. Mayer KH, Agwu A, Malebranche D. Barriers to the wider use of pre-exposure prophylaxis in the United States: a narrative review. *Adv Ther.* 2020;37(5):1778–1811. https://doi.org/10.1007/s12325-020-01295-0
21. Barry V, Dasgupta S, Weller DL, et al. Patterns in COVID-19 vaccination coverage, by social vulnerability and urbanicity—United States, December 14, 2020–May 1, 2021. *MMWR Morb Mortal Wkly Rep.* 2021;70(22):818–824. https://doi.org/10.15585/mmwr.mm7022e1
22. Crenshaw K. Mapping the margins: intersectionality, identity politics, and violence against women of color. *Stanford Law Rev.* 1990;43(6):1241–1299. https://doi.org/10.2307/1229039
23. Bowleg L. Evolving intersectionality within public health: from analysis to action. *Am J Public Health.* 2021;111(1):88–90. https://doi.org/10.2105/AJPH.2020.306031
24. Hankivsky O, Christoffersen A. Intersectionality and the determinants of health: a Canadian perspective. *Crit Public Health.* 2008;18(3):271–283. https://doi.org/10.1080/09581590802294296
25. Tobin-Tyler E, Teitelbaum JB. *Essentials of Health Justice: Law, Policy, and Structural Change.* 2018. Google Books. Available at: https://books.google.com/books?hl=en&lr=&id=dit4EAAAQBAJ&oi=fnd&pg=PT17&dq=%22Essentials+of+Health+Justice:+A+Primer%22+through+APHA+&ots=x68X-OH-_V&sig=fNrS8ZyHfZh8Y21ltT9_ZUoKLL4#v=onepage&q&f=false. Accessed July 6, 2022.
26. Schneider MJ. *Introduction to Public Health.* Google Books. 2020. Available at: https://books.google.co.uk/books?hl=en&lr=&id=Of_2DwAAQBAJ&oi=fnd&pg=PP1&dq=what+is+public+health+&ots=-JgJYPfvo9&sig=w2TYtMxYbRZEAboFf7LeEhRCfQs#v=onepage&q=whatispublichealth&f=false. Accessed December 17, 2021.
27. Kaba M. *We Do This' Til We Free Us: Abolitionist Organizing and Transforming Justice.* Chicago, IL: Haymarket Books; 2021.
28. Douglas JA, Grills C, Villanueva S, Subica AM. Empowerment praxis: community organizing to redress systemic health disparities. *Am J Community Psychol.* 2016;58(3-4):488–498. https://doi.org/10.1002/ajcp.12101
29. Pastor M, Terriquez V, Lin M. How community organizing promotes health equity, and how health equity affects organizing. *Health Aff (Millwood).* 2018;37(3):358–363. https://doi.org/101377/hlthaff20171285
30. The White House. National COVID-19 preparedness plan. March 2022. Available at: https://www.whitehouse.gov/wp-content/uploads/2022/03/NAT-COVID-19-PREPAREDNESS-PLAN.pdf. Accessed December 17, 2021.
31. Centers for Disease Control and Prevention. The 10 essential public health services. 2020. Available at: https://phnci.org/uploads/resource-files/EPHS-English.pdf. Accessed September 29, 2020.
32. Mohr RD. AIDS, gays, and state coercion. *Bioethics.* 1987;1(1):35–50. https://doi.org/10.1111/j.1467-8519.1987.tb00003.x
33. Scoville C, McCumber A, Amironesei R, Jeon J. Mask refusal backlash: the politicization of face masks in the American public sphere during the early stages of the COVID-19 pandemic. *Socius.* 2022;8:1–22. https://doi.org/10.1177/23780231221093158
34. Callard F, Perego E. How and why patients made long COVID. *Soc Sci Med.* 2021;268:113426. https://doi.org/10.1016/j.socscimed.2020.113426
35. Cowan H. Taking the National(ism) out of the National Health Service: re-locating agency to amongst ourselves. *Crit Public Health.* 2021;31(2):134–143. https://doi.org/10.1080/09581596.2020.1836328
36. Campbell C, Cornish F. Public health activism in changing times: re-locating collective agency. *Crit Public Health.* 2021;31(2):125–133. https://doi.org/10.1080/09581596.2021.1878110
37. Taylor K. The emerging movement for police and prison abolition. *The New Yorker.* May 7, 2021. Available at: https://www.newyorker.com/news/our-columnists/the-emerging-movement-for-police-and-prison-abolition. Accessed July 6, 2022.
38. Hoffman B. Health care reform and social movements in the United States. *Am J Public Health.* 2008;98(suppl 1):S69–S79. https://doi.org/10.2105/AJPH.98.Supplement_1.S69

Medication Abortion "Reversal" Laws: How Unsound Science Paved the Way for Dangerous Abortion Policy

Sara K. Redd, PhD, MSPH, Roula AbiSamra, MPH, Sarah C. Blake, PhD, MA, Kelli A. Komro, PhD, MPH, Rachel Neal, MD, Whitney S. Rice, DrPH, MPH, and Kelli S. Hall, PhD, MS

See also Skuster, p. 138.

Objectives. To longitudinally examine the legal landscape of laws requiring abortion patients be informed about the possibility of medication abortion (MAB) "reversal" (in quotes as it does not refer to an evidence-based medical procedure).

Methods. We collected legal data on enacted state MAB-reversal laws across all 50 US states and Washington, DC, (collectively, states) from 2012 through 2021. We descriptively analyzed these laws to identify legal variation over time and geography, and conducted a content analysis to identify qualitative themes and patterns in MAB-reversal laws.

Results. As of 2021, 14 states (27%)—mostly in the midwestern and southern United States—have enacted MAB-reversal laws. States largely use explicit language to describe reversal, require patients receive information during preabortion counseling, require physicians or physicians' agents to inform patients, instruct patients to contact a health care provider or visit "abortion pill reversal" resources for more information, and require reversal information be posted on state-managed Web sites.

Conclusions. Reversal laws continue a dangerous precedent of using unsound science to justify laws regulating abortion access, intrude upon the patient–provider relationship, and may negatively affect the emotional and physical health of patients seeking an MAB. (*Am J Public Health*. 2023;113(2):202–212. https://doi.org/10.2105/AJPH.2022.307140)

AJPH February 2023, Vol 113, No. 2

Medication abortion (MAB)—the use of medications to induce an abortion up to the first 10 to 11 weeks of pregnancy—has rapidly become a popular abortion care method over the past 2 decades. While abortions in the United States have largely decreased since 2000, MABs have continued to rise and currently constitute the majority of all abortions in the United States, accounting for 54% of all nonhospital abortions as of 2020.[1] In addition, MAB is highly effective and extraordinarily safe, with a less-than-1% risk of complications.[1] With its rise in popularity, MAB has become a frequent target for state legislatures seeking to restrict abortion access and provision. One such regulation is MAB "reversal" laws ("reversal" placed in quotations, as this term does not refer to an evidence-based medical procedure), which—like other biased abortion counseling laws—require that patients receive medically inaccurate information about the possibility of reversing a MAB.

Fewer than 0.005% of patients who use mifepristone choose to continue their pregnancy; the current clinical recommendation for such patients is watchful waiting and fetal monitoring.[2] MAB reversal is an experimental procedure involving the administration of a high dose of progesterone following the initial dose of mifepristone should a patient who is using MAB choose to continue their pregnancy. MAB reversal was initially described in a 2012 case series by Delgado and Davenport, which presented cases of 6 patients who received 200 milligrams of progesterone following mifepristone ingestion, 4 of whom carried pregnancies to term.[3] Based on this 2012 case series, a 2017 article by Garratt and Turner detailed cases of 3 patients treated with progesterone following mifepristone ingestion, 2 of whom carried pregnancies to term.[4] The following year, Delgado et al. published a second case series of 754 patients who underwent the experimental procedure, reporting an "overall rate of reversal of mifepristone [of] 48%."[5]

Numerous ethical and scientific problems highlight the poor quality of these case series. The lack of evident oversight by an institutional review board or ethics committee and apparent failure to obtain patient consent demonstrate neglect of common ethical standards and study participant protection. Scientifically, the data produced by these studies are of a low standard because of the failure to employ standardized scientific protocols, lack of comparison group, artificial inflation of pregnancy completion rates by assessing pregnancy viability before reversal, and incomplete reporting of patient outcomes. Together, these studies fail to provide rigorous scientific evidence supporting MAB reversal.[2]

One randomized clinical trial attempted to evaluate safety and efficacy of MAB reversal[6] but was ceased prematurely to protect participants because of 3 instances of severe hemorrhage requiring ambulance hospital transport. Study authors concluded that MAB reversal is "experimental and should be offered only in institutional review board-approved human clinical trials to ensure proper oversight."[6(p164)] Experts from the medical and public health communities have denounced MAB reversal as unsafe, unproven, and unethical.[6–10] However, MAB reversal swiftly gained the attention of state legislators, who have subsequently enacted legislation requiring MAB reversal information be included during the abortion process.

A summary by Bhatti et al. described state MAB-reversal legislation as of 2018, noting that legislators had introduced MAB-reversal bills in 9 states and successfully enacted laws in 3 of those states.[9] Given the continued increase in antiabortion legislation—including MAB-reversal laws—since 2018, we collected data on state MAB-reversal laws through 2021 to provide an updated overview of the MAB-reversal legal landscape in the United States. We descriptively analyzed these laws to identify legal variation over time and geography and conducted a content analysis[11] of legal texts to identify themes and patterns in MAB-reversal laws.

METHODS

We collected data on MAB-reversal laws across all 50 states and Washington, DC, (collectively, states) from 2012 to 2021. We gathered state statutory laws requiring patients be told about MAB reversal during the abortion process, including via conversations with clinic providers or staff, physical signs, discharge materials, medication guides, or state-managed Web sites. We included laws currently in effect and temporarily enjoined pending litigation and tracked implementation from January 1, 2012, through December 31, 2021. We gathered full versions of legal text using Nexis Uni and validated our data using LawAtlas's Medication Abortion Requirements data set.[12] We reported the number and percentage of states with enacted MAB-reversal laws for each year of the study period to examine their proliferation over the study period. To visualize these time trends, we created a map indicating the year in which each state enacted the first reversal law.

In addition, we conducted a content analysis of statutes,[11] identifying themes and patterns in how states prescribe MAB-reversal information be provided to patients. To conduct the content analysis, we first created a tentative set of coding categories based on a preliminary examination of the MAB-reversal legal data, which we refined following an in-depth review of the data. Codes examined the following domains: language used to describe reversal (i.e., explicit vs generic language); reference to supporting "scientific research"; when, how, and by whom patients are informed; what actions patients should take; penalties for providers or clinics; and requirements for information on state-managed Web sites. We then applied the refined codes to the data, ensuring objectivity and reliability through repeated coding of the laws by the coder. We then summarized coding findings (e.g., documenting the recurrence of themes present in the laws) and reported them in a systematic manner.

RESULTS

Table 1 displays a list of states with MAB-reversal laws, corresponding legal citation, legislation, enactment and effective dates, and current status of each law.

Medication Abortion Reversal Law Variation

As of December 31, 2021, 14 states (27%) had MAB-reversal laws enacted. Following publication of Delgado and Davenport's 2012 case series,[3] the first reversal laws were enacted in Arizona and Arkansas in 2015, although Arizona's 2015 reversal law—which contained explicit references to "reversal"—was repealed and replaced in 2016 with

TABLE 1— State Medication Abortion–Reversal Laws by Legal Citation, Corresponding Legislation, Enactment and Effective Dates, and Current Law Status: United States, 2012–2021

State	Legal Citation	Corresponding Legislation	Enactment Date	Effective Date	Current Status
AZ	Ariz Rev Stat §36-2153	2015 Ariz SB 1318 2016 Ariz SB 1112	Mar 30, 2015 May 17, 2016	Jul 3, 2015 Aug 6, 2016	Effective
AR	Ark Code Ann §20-16-1703 Ark Code Ann §20-16-1704	2015 Ark HB 1578	Apr 6, 2015	Jul 22, 2015	Effective
ID	Idaho Code §18-609	2018 Idaho SB 1243	Mar 20, 2018	Jul 1, 2018	Effective
IN	Ind Code Ann §1-34-2-1	2021 Ind HEA 1577	Apr 29, 2021	Jul 1, 2021	Enjoined—preliminary injunction granted Jun 30, 2021
KY	Ky Rev Stat §311.725 Ky Rev Stat §311.774	2019 Ky SB 50	Mar 26, 2019	Jun 27, 2019	Effective
LA	La Rev Stat §40:1061.11.1	2021 La HB 578	Jun 19, 2021	Aug 1, 2021	Effective
MT	Mont Code Ann 50-20-707 Mont Code Ann 50-20-708	2021 Mont HB 171	Apr 26, 2021	Oct 1, 2021	Effective
NE	Neb Rev Stat §28-327 Neb Rev Stat §28-327.01	2019 Neb LB 209	Jun 4, 2019	Sep 1, 2019	Effective
ND	ND Cent Code, §14-02.1-02 ND Cent Code, §14-02.1-02.1	2019 ND HB 1336	Mar 22, 2019	Aug 1, 2019	Enjoined—preliminary injunction granted Sep 10, 2019
OK	63 Okla Stat §1-756	2019 Okla SB 614	Apr 25, 2019	Nov 1, 2019	Enjoined—temporary injunction granted Oct 25, 2019
SD	SD Codified Laws §34-23A-10.1 SD Codified Laws §34-23A-10.4	2016 SD HB 1157 2021 SD HB 1130	Mar 16, 2016 Mar 25, 2021	Jul 1, 2016, Jul 1, 2021	Effective
TN	Tenn Code Ann §39-15-218	2019 Tenn HB 2263	Jul 13, 2020	Oct 1, 2020	Enjoined—temporary restraining order granted Sep 29, 2020
UT	Utah Code Ann §76-7-305 Utah Code Ann §76-7-305.5	Abortion Law Amendments, 2018 Utah SB 118	Mar 19, 2018	May 8, 2018	Effective
WV	W Va Code §16-2I-2 W Va Code §16-2I-3 W Va Code §16-2I-4	2021 W Va HB 2982	Apr 28, 2021	Jul 9, 2021	Effective

more generic reversal language following backlash from constituents. Over the next 6 years, 12 additional states enacted MAB-reversal laws. Following Arizona and Arkansas, South Dakota enacted its reversal law in 2016, followed by Idaho and Utah in 2018.

Following the 2018 publication by Delgado et al.,[5] the number of states enacting MAB-reversal laws increased notably. In 2019, Kentucky, Nebraska, North Dakota, and Oklahoma enacted reversal laws, and Tennessee enacted its reversal law in 2020. Lastly, in 2021, 4 additional states—Indiana, Louisiana, Montana, and West Virginia—enacted reversal laws. Of the 14 states with enacted MAB-reversal laws as of December 31, 2021, 10 of these states—Arizona, Arkansas, Idaho, Kentucky, Louisiana, Montana, Nebraska, South Dakota, Utah, and West Virginia—had laws in effect. The remaining 4 states—Indiana, North Dakota, Oklahoma, and Tennessee—had laws that were temporarily enjoined pending litigation. Geographically (Figure 1), 6 of the 14 states (43%) were located in the South (Arkansas, Kentucky, Louisiana, Oklahoma, Tennessee, and West Virginia), 4 (29%) in the Midwest (Indiana, Nebraska, North Dakota, and South Dakota), and 4 (29%) in the West (Arizona, Idaho, Montana, and Utah).

Content Analysis

Tables 2 and 3 display content analysis results regarding the following themes: language describing "reversal"; references to supporting "scientific research"; when, how, and by whom patients are informed; patient actions; penalties for providers or clinics; and state Web site requirements.

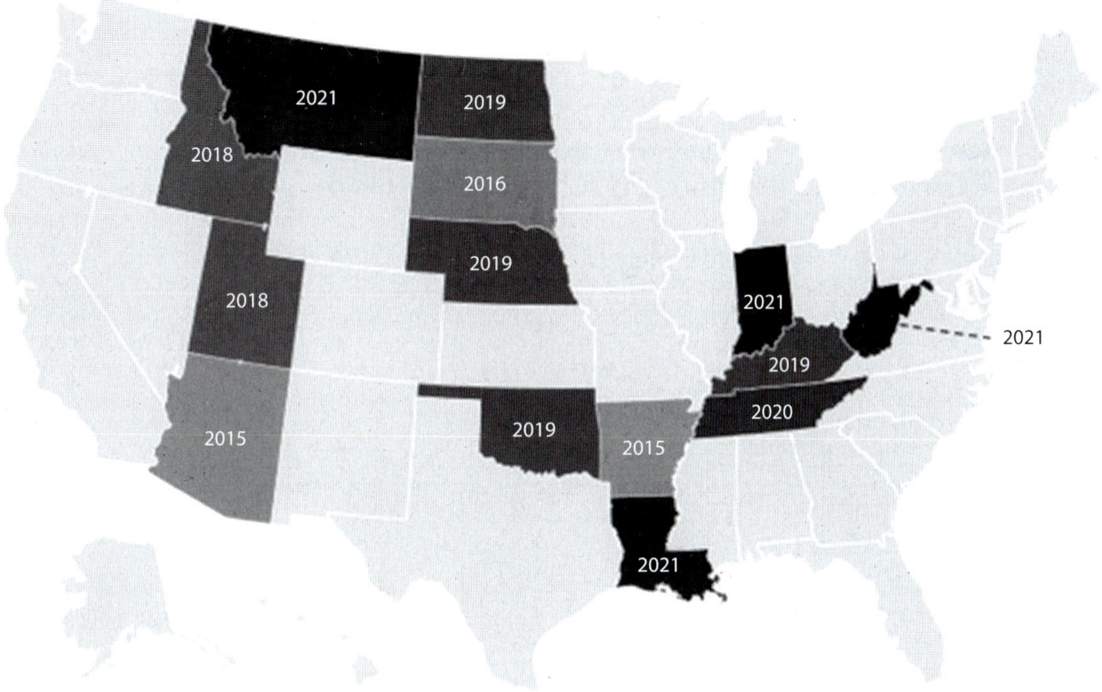

Year	State Abbreviations	No. (%)
2012–2014	-	0 (0)
2015	AZ, AR	2 (4)
2016	AZ, AR, SD	3 (6)
2017	AZ, AR, SD	3 (6)
2018	AZ, AR, ID, SD, UT	5 (10)
2019	AZ, AR, ID, KY, NE, ND, OK, SD, UT	9 (18)
2020	AZ, AR, ID, KY, NE, ND, OK, SD, TN, UT	10 (20)
2021	AZ, AR, ID, IN, KY, LA, MT, NE, ND, OK, SD, TN, UT, WV	14 (27)

FIGURE 1— States With Enacted Medication Abortion–Reversal Laws by Year First Law Enacted and Incidence by Year: United States, 2012–2021

Reversal language. We first categorized type of language used to describe MAB reversal as either explicit (e.g., "the effects of mifepristone can be reversed") or generic (e.g., "mifepristone is not always effective"). Eight states' laws make explicit references to reversal, stating that MABs can be reversed. For instance, Arkansas's law states a physician must inform the patient of "information on reversing the effects of abortion-inducing drugs."[13] Six states' laws do not specifically mention iterations of the word "reversal," instead using generic language to imply that MABs can be reversed, as in West Virginia's law: "it may be possible to counteract the intended effects of a mifepristone chemical abortion."[14]

Reference to scientific evidence or research. Although most states refrain from referencing scientific evidence, 5 include references to research in the laws. Of note, 4 of the 5 laws referencing research were enacted after the 2018 Delgado et al. publication.[5] Tennessee's law states, "recent research has indicated that mifepristone alone is not always effective in ending a pregnancy."[15] Indiana's law appears to reference the mixed evidence base around reversal, noting,

> some [emphasis added] evidence suggests that the effects of Mifepristone may be avoided, ceased, or reversed if the second pill, Misoprostol, has not been taken.[16]

AJPH February 2023, Vol 113, No. 2

TABLE 2— State Medication Abortion-Reversal Law Content Analysis—Language, Research, and When and How Patients Are Informed: United States, 2012–2021

State	Reversal Language	References Research	When Are Patients Informed?	How Are Patients Informed?
AZ	Generic language: "the use of mifepristone alone to end a pregnancy is not always effective."	No	Upon patient contacting clinic	Not specified
AR	Explicit language: "It may be possible to reverse [Mifepristone's] intended effect."	No	Preabortion counseling At discharge	Orally, in person (preabortion counseling) In writing (discharge materials)
ID	Explicit language: "interventions, if any, that may affect . . . the reversal of a chemical abortion."	No	Preabortion counseling	In writing
IN	Explicit language: "the effects of Mifepristone may be avoided, ceased, or reversed."	Yes: "Some evidence suggests . . ."	Preabortion counseling At discharge	Orally, in person (preabortion counseling) In writing (discharge materials)
KY	Explicit language: "to reverse the effects of prescription drugs intended to induce abortion."	No	Preabortion counseling Receipt of prescription	Orally, not specified (preabortion counseling) In writing (with prescription)
LA	Generic language: "the first pill, . . . mifepristone, is not always effective in ending a pregnancy."	Yes: "Research has indicated . . ."	At discharge Receipt of prescription	In writing
MT	Explicit language: "reversing the effects of abortion-inducing drugs."	No	Preabortion counseling	In writing
NE	Generic language: "mifepristone alone is not always effective in ending a pregnancy."	Yes: "Research indicates . . ."	Preabortion counseling	Orally, in person or over telephone
ND	Explicit language: "it may be possible to reverse the effects of an abortion-inducing drug."	No	Preabortion counseling	Not specified
OK	Explicit language: "Mifepristone . . . alone is not always effective in ending a pregnancy. It may be possible to reverse its intended effect."	No	Preabortion counseling Upon physical visit to clinic (clinic signs) At discharge	Orally, in person or over telephone (preabortion counseling) In writing (clinic signs, discharge materials)
SD	Generic language: "it is still possible to discontinue a drug-induced abortion."	No	Preabortion counseling At discharge	In writing
TN	Explicit language: "It may be possible to avoid, cease, or even reverse the intended effects of a chemical abortion utilizing mifepristone."	Yes: "Recent developing research has indicated . . ."	Preabortion counseling Upon physical visit to clinic (clinic signs) At discharge	Not specified (preabortion counseling) In writing (clinic signs, discharge materials)
UT	Generic language: "aborting a medication-induced abortion."	Yes: "Research indicates . . ."	Preabortion counseling At discharge	Orally, in-person (preabortion counseling) In writing (discharge materials)
WV	Generic language: "it may be possible to counteract the intended effects of a mifepristone chemical abortion."	No	Preabortion counseling At discharge	Orally, in person or via telephone (preabortion counseling) In writing (discharge materials)

TABLE 3— State Medication Abortion-Reversal Law Content Analysis—Who Informs Patients, Patient Actions, Penalties, and Web Site Requirements: United States, 2012–2021

State	Who Informs Patients?	What Actions Should Patients Take?	Penalty for Provider or Clinic?	Web Site Requirement?
AZ	Clinic staff	Contact physician	None specified	Yes
AR	Health care professional (physician or physician's agent)	Search "abortion pill reversal" online	None specified	Yes
ID	Health care professional (physician or physician's agent)	Contact health care provider	None specified	Yes
IN	Health care professional (physician)	Visit "abortion pill reversal" Web site or call hotline	None specified	None specified
KY	Health care professional (physician, licensed nurse, PA, or social worker)	Contact physician	Provider penalty: denial, probation, suspension, or revocation of license	None specified
LA	Health care professional (physician or physician's agent)	Contact physician or health care provider	None specified	None specified
MT	Health care professional	Visit "abortion pill reversal" Web site or call hotline	None specified	None specified
NE	Health care professional (physician or PA or RN as physician's agent)	Visit state Web site	None specified	Yes
ND	Health care professional (physician or physician's agent)	Contact health care provider	None specified	Yes
OK	Health care professional (physician or physician's agent; preabortion counseling and discharge materials) Clinic (sign in clinic)	Visit "abortion pill reversal" Web site or call hotline	Financial penalty for clinic or facility	Yes
SD	Health care professional (physician)	Visit state Web site or contact health care provider	None specified	Yes
TN	Health care professional (physician; preabortion counseling) Health care professional (physician or physician's agent; discharge materials) Clinic (sign in clinic)	Visit state Web site or contact health care provider	Financial penalty for clinic or facility	Yes
UT	Clinic or hospital staff or health care professional (physician, RN, NP, APRN, CNM, genetic counselor, or PA)	Contact physician	Provider penalty: suspension or revocation of license, administrative penalties	Yes
WV	Health care professional (physician or physician's agent; preabortion counseling and discharge materials)	Contact physician	None specified	Yes

Note. APRN = advanced-practice registered nurse; CNM = certified nurse midwife; NP = nurse practitioner; PA = physician's assistant; RN = registered nurse.

When patients are informed. In 12 of the 14 states with MAB-reversal laws, patients must be informed about the possibility of reversal during preabortion counseling. Many states require providers or staff to counsel patients at multiple points throughout the abortion care process, such as during preabortion counseling and at discharge. Seven states require informing patients during preabortion counseling and at discharge, and 1 state (Kentucky) requires informing patients during preabortion counseling and upon receipt of the prescription. Two states—Oklahoma and Tennessee—require clinics to post visible signs in the clinic, passively informing patients upon clinic entrance. Both laws are presently enjoined and, thus, not in effect.

Two states require informing patients at unique points in the abortion care process. In Louisiana, providers must inform patients either at discharge or upon receipt of their prescription, via the following:

(1) Stapling the disclosure statement to a bag, envelope, or other package that contains misoprostol for the [patient] to self-administer at home.
(2) Attaching the disclosure statement to a written prescription for misoprostol provided by the physician or the person acting under the physician's direction.
(3) Attaching the disclosure statement to the patient's discharge instructions if the prescription for misoprostol is sent directly to a pharmacy.[17]

In Arizona, patients are informed only in the specific circumstance in which a patient who has taken mifepristone, but not misoprostol, contacts an abortion clinic

> questioning her decision to terminate her pregnancy or seeking information regarding the health of her fetus or the efficacy of mifepristone alone to terminate a pregnancy.[18]

How patients are informed. Twelve states specify that patients should be informed using written or oral communication. Of those 12 states, 11 states require patients be informed in writing during preabortion counseling, at discharge, upon receipt of prescription, or via clinic signs. Seven states require that patients receive the information orally during preabortion counseling, with 6 states requiring in-person or offering the option of in-person or over the phone. Although Kentucky specifies that patients should be informed orally, the law does not specify whether oral communication must be in-person or over the phone. Two states—Arizona and North Dakota—do not specify the way patients are to be informed.

Who informs patients. In 13 states, MAB-reversal laws specify that health care professionals—namely, a physician or advanced practice clinician acting as a physician's agent—inform patients of the possibility of reversal. While some states, such as West Virginia, specify a "physician or physician's agent,"[14] other states, such as Kentucky, detail the other medical professionals to whom the law may apply: "a physician, licensed nurse, physician assistant, or social worker to whom the responsibility has been delegated by the physician."[19] Tennessee's law requires a physician to inform patients during preabortion counseling, while a physician or physician's agent reminds patients when providing discharge materials.

Two states—Arizona and Utah—delineate clinic staff as an informing party; Arizona's law identifies clinic staff as the party who informs patients (i.e., "the abortion clinic staff"),[18] while Utah's lists clinic or hospital staff as 1 potential party who might inform patients, along with a physician or physician's agent (i.e., "a staff member of an abortion clinic or hospital, physician, registered nurse, nurse practitioner, advanced practice registered nurse, certified nurse midwife, genetic counselor, or physician's assistant").[20] Lastly, 2 states—Oklahoma and Tennessee—include clinics as an informing party via in-clinic signs (both laws were enjoined at the time of our study). Oklahoma's law states,

> Any private office, freestanding outpatient clinic, hospital or other facility or clinic in which medication abortions . . . are provided shall conspicuously post a sign . . . so as to be clearly visible to patients.[21]

What actions patients should take. Nine states instruct patients to contact a physician or health care provider for additional information, sometimes noting to patients that "time is of the essence." Three states instruct patients to visit a state-managed Web site to gain access to "abortion pill reversal" information services, including a Web site (https://www.abortionpillreversal.com) and telephone hotline run by the Abortion Pill Rescue Network at Heartbeat International, a large international antiabortion organization. For example, Nebraska's law states, "information on finding immediate medical assistance is available on the web site of the Department of Health and Human Services"[22]; upon visiting this Web site, visitors are directed to the "abortion pill reversal" telephone hotline. An additional 3 states instruct patients to contact "abortion pill reversal" information services and provide the contact information directly, such as in Montana's law, which states:

> Information on the potential ability of qualified medical practitioners to reverse the effects of an abortion obtained through the use of abortion-inducing drugs is available at www.abortionpillreversal.com, or you can contact (877) 558-0333 for assistance in locating a medical professional who can aid in the reversal of an abortion.[23]

Finally, 1 state—Arkansas—instructs patients to "search 'abortion pill reversal' online."[13]

Provider or clinic penalties. Four states include specific penalties for providers or clinics offering abortion services that do not comply with MAB-reversal laws. Two states, Kentucky and Utah, detail penalties for individual providers who do not comply with the reversal law, including denial, probation, suspension, or revocation of a provider's medical license or administrative penalties. Two additional states, Oklahoma and Tennessee, specify financial penalties for clinics that fail to comply with the reversal law. In Tennessee, any

> facility or clinic that negligently fails to post a sign . . . [shall receive] a civil penalty of ten thousand dollars ($10,000). Each day on which an abortion . . . is performed . . . during which the required sign is not posted is a separate violation.[15]

State-managed Web sites. Lastly, 10 states require that state departments of health develop and maintain public Web sites providing an online version of preabortion counseling materials, including reversal information. Laws in the remaining 4 states do not specify a Web site requirement.

DISCUSSION

Following the initial 2012 publication on MAB reversal,[3] the number of states with MAB-reversal laws enacted grew from zero in 2012 to 14 in 2021. The largest annual changes in laws occurred in 2019 and 2021, following the 2018 publication by Delgado et al.,[5] during which 4 states enacted MAB-reversal laws. Ten of the 14 states with reversal laws are in the Midwest or South, regions of the country with the most restrictive environments toward abortion.[24,25] Content analysis revealed that state laws often use explicit language detailing the possibility of reversal and require information be provided to patients orally or in writing during preabortion counseling or at discharge, usually by a physician or physician's agent. State laws largely instruct patients to contact a health care provider for more information on reversal or to visit an "abortion pill reversal" Web site and telephone hotline, and require that a state agency post information about reversal on a state-managed Web site.

Public policy scholar Paul Cairney proffers that policymakers rely on rational and irrational solutions to make policy decisions, balancing the prioritization of certain sources of information ("rational solutions") with emotions, gut feelings, beliefs, and habits ("irrational sources").[26] In the case of MAB reversal, antiabortion legislators employ both rational and irrational sources when enacting these policies, combining the rational source of Delgado's and others' work on MAB reversal with their own "irrational" antiabortion beliefs. In addition, antiabortion advocates and lobbyists have made and will continue to make concerted efforts to rally policymakers to enact reversal legislation. Groups such as the National Right to Life Committee, which actively advocate for restrictive antiabortion legislation, have named MAB-reversal laws as one of their key legislative targets. The relatively swift proliferation of MAB-reversal laws in US states highlights the increasing efforts at the state legislative level to restrict abortion access and the tendency for policymakers to ground antiabortion policy in moral and religious arguments[27] and support from antiabortion activists, despite positive public support for abortion access remaining steady.[27–30]

On June 24, 2022, the Supreme Court of the United States overturned the constitutional right to an abortion established in *Roe v. Wade* in their ruling on *Dobbs v. Jackson Women's Health Organization*. As of September 30, 2022, of the 14 states with MAB-reversal laws, 7—Arkansas, Indiana, Kentucky, Louisiana, Oklahoma, South Dakota, and Tennessee—have banned all abortions, with very limited exceptions.[31] Four additional states—Arizona, North Dakota, Utah, and West Virginia—have either pre-*Roe* bans or trigger bans that are currently enjoined and, thus, not in effect.[31] Abortion remains legal in the remaining 3 states—Idaho, Montana, and Nebraska—although state environments are changing rapidly and could shift at any time.

The post-*Dobbs* landscape has shifted the importance of MAB-reversal laws considerably. In states with complete bans in effect, clinicians are unable to prescribe mifepristone or misoprostol for a MAB, thus rendering MAB-reversal laws moot. Exceptions to these complete bans are extremely limited, with states typically allowing abortions only to save the pregnant person's life[31]—a scenario in which an abortion would likely be procedural rather than medical. However, in the 4 states with abortion bans that are currently enjoined and not in effect, or in the 3 states where abortion remains legal, MAB-reversal laws remain significant.

Furthermore, in states that have not yet enacted or do not have the legislative capacity to enact total bans, or in states that have begun or are expected to receive a surge of out-of-state patients, MAB-reversal laws will likely become increasingly important mechanisms for antiabortion policymakers. For instance, at least 3 additional states (Georgia, Iowa, and Maryland) introduced MAB-reversal laws during the pre-*Dobbs* 2022 legislative session. These trends, along with the increasing fervor of antiabortion legislators and advocates to eliminate abortion access, suggest that MAB-reversal laws are an important player in the antiabortion policymaking agenda that will continue to appear in future legislative sessions.

Implications for Patients, Practice, and Policymaking

Our findings have important implications for the health of patients, providers, the patient–provider relationship, and policymaking, particularly in this post-*Dobbs* era. Regarding patients, MAB-reversal policies have the potential to increase stigma and shame around receiving an abortion, decrease patient empowerment and self-efficacy, and make patients vulnerable to physical complications.

First, reversal policies are rooted in abortion stigma.[32] Use of language referencing the possibility to "reverse," "correct," or "counteract" the effects of mifepristone conveys the idea that choosing a MAB is a mistake—although people seeking abortions have high degrees of certainty about their decisions[33–35]—and, therefore, lawmakers are giving patients an opportunity to correct their error. Abortion stigma leads to experiences of stress, shame, and guilt among abortion patients, resulting in reduced self-efficacy around decision-making, decreased perceptions of social support, and increased psychological distress.[36,37]

Second, some states instruct patients interested in reversal to visit the "abortion pill reversal" Web site run by the Abortion Pill Rescue Network at Heartbeat International, an international antiabortion association that reportedly supports the largest network of crisis pregnancy centers—antiabortion organizations posing as health care clinics that attempt to dissuade people from considering abortion[38]—in the world. This Web site and its associated hotline use coercive, antiabortion messaging (e.g., "Time is precious, and so is your baby—call us today"; "We are the agile guardians of that precious moment in time when a woman chooses to give her unborn child a chance to fight for life") to transmit misinformation about the possibility and evidence behind reversal. Further exposure to misinformation and stigmatizing messaging may reduce patient self-efficacy and increase experiences of shame or guilt around their decision,[39] which may increase a patient's drive to pursue reversal.

Third, MAB-reversal laws in 10 states require publication of information about MAB reversal, along with other biased statements about abortion, on state department of health Web sites. State departments of health are generally perceived by the public to be trusted sources of information for public health and health promotion[40]; thus, state-sanctioned promotion of abortion misinformation has great potential to mislead and endanger the public. Requiring promotion of medically inaccurate information such as MAB reversal compromises the integrity of entities with a mission to promote and protect the public's health.

Lastly, MAB reversal may result in increased risk of physical complications, including severe hemorrhage. As Creinin et al. assert,

> patients who use mifepristone for a medical abortion should be advised that not using misoprostol could result in severe hemorrhage, even with progesterone treatment.[6(p162)]

Poor outcomes following MAB reversal have the potential to negatively affect the health and well-being of patients seeking a MAB, particularly those who are Black, other people of color, or those of lower socioeconomic status, groups that are disproportionately affected by restrictive abortion policies and experience the highest maternal mortality rates.[41–44]

In addition, this study has important implications for provider practice and the patient–provider relationship. MAB-reversal laws are another example of legislation requiring clinicians to transmit misinformation to their patients. Many states require inclusion of other inaccurate or misleading information in preabortion counseling, such as inaccurate statements about mental health effects of having an abortion, fetal pain, or purported links between receiving an abortion and breast cancer.[45] These laws are burdensome to providers; interfere with their ability to provide comprehensive, patient-centered care[46]; violate the accepted standards of informed consent; and negatively affect the trust and rapport of the patient–provider relationship.[47] Although MAB-reversal laws similarly intrude on and undermine the patient–provider relationship, they further jeopardize the role of provider as healer and violate medical ethics by requiring providers to impart information about an experimental procedure that may cause patients harm.

Finally, study findings have clear implications for the post-*Dobbs* policymaking sphere. MAB-reversal laws reflect the general trend for antiabortion policy to be grounded in unsound science and to promote misinformation. As noted earlier, MAB-reversal laws will likely become increasingly popular among antiabortion policymakers and advocates seeking to restrict abortion to the greatest extent possible, particularly in states without total abortion bans. When opposing enactment of additional MAB-reversal laws and leading efforts to repeal existing reversal laws, policymakers should focus on the weak scientific evidence behind these policies, partnering with clinicians and researchers to debunk the science. Furthermore, policymakers should collaborate with community members, organizations, advocates, clinicians, and researchers to promote egalitarian policymaking grounded in high-quality evidence and person-centered research around abortion, which centers the communities traditionally left out of policymaking.

Limitations

There are some limitations to our analysis. First, the inclusion of enjoined laws in this analysis may artificially inflate the prevalence of MAB-reversal regulation in the United States. However, because policy implementation is often ambiguous and enjoined laws may influence patient and provider beliefs and experiences, their inclusion was important to this analysis. Second, the laws reviewed here do not reflect the implementation or enforcement of these policies, which may vary from how laws are written; thus, we can only infer how these laws influence provider practice and patient experiences. Third, this analysis focused only on enacted legislation; it does not capture legislation that was introduced in but not enacted by a state legislature. Thus, this analysis does not fully reflect the frequency with which MAB-reversal legislation was introduced into state legislatures.

Conclusions

In this analysis, we critically examined an understudied and dangerous means by which state legislators regulate abortion. We explored the path between scientific evidence and policymaking, highlighting a case in which sensationalized research, denounced as unsafe and of low quality by experts, nevertheless quickly inspired state antiabortion legislation, requiring the transmission of medically inaccurate information to patients. Our findings highlight the rapid proliferation of MAB-reversal laws and the various ways in which states regulate informing patients about reversal. Findings from this study can provide evidence for the concerning relationship between antiabortion science and policymaking, stimulate further rigorous research of historical legal data, and inform abortion policymaking, including the repealing of MAB-reversal laws. AJPH

ABOUT THE AUTHORS

Sara K. Redd and Sarah C. Blake are with the Department of Health Policy and Management, Rollins School of Public Health, Emory University, Atlanta, GA. Roula AbiSamra is with the Amplify Georgia Collaborative, Atlanta. Kelli A. Komro and Whitney S. Rice are with the Department of Behavioral, Social, and Health Education Sciences, Rollins School of Public Health. Rachel Neal is with the Department of Gynecology and Obstetrics, School of Medicine, Emory University. Kelli S. Hall is with the Heilbrunn Department of Population and Family Health, Mailman School of Public Health, Columbia University, New York, NY.

CORRESPONDENCE

Correspondence should be sent to Sara K. Redd, Department of Health Policy and Management, Rollins School of Public Health, Emory University, 1518 Clifton Rd NE, Atlanta, GA 30322 (e-mail: skredd@emory.edu). Reprints can be ordered at https://ajph.org by clicking the "Reprints" link.

PUBLICATION INFORMATION

Full Citation: Redd SK, AbiSamra R, Blake SC, et al. Medication abortion "reversal" laws: how unsound science paved the way for dangerous abortion policy. *Am J Public Health*. 2023;113(2):202–212.

Acceptance Date: September 28, 2022.

DOI: https://doi.org/10.2105/AJPH.2022.307140

CONTRIBUTORS

S. K. Redd, S. C. Blake, K. A. Komro, W. S. Rice, and K. S. Hall conceptualized and designed the study. S. K. Redd collected data, completed analyses, interpreted findings, and led article writing. R. AbiSamra, S. C. Blake, K. A. Komro, R. Neal, W. S. Rice, and K. S. Hall assisted with interpretation of findings and article writing and provided critical feedback on the article. All authors contributed to the article and approved the submitted version.

ACKNOWLEDGMENTS

S. K. Redd was funded in part by the Center for Reproductive Health Research in the Southeast (RISE).

We acknowledge Erica Reeves, JD, from Akin Gump Strauss Hauer and Feld LLP, Washington, DC, who provided research assistance on a previous iteration of this study during her time at Emory University School of Law.

CONFLICTS OF INTEREST

The authors have no conflicts of interest to disclose.

HUMAN PARTICIPANT PROTECTION

This research did not require institutional review board review as it did not involve human participants.

REFERENCES

1. Jones RK, Nash E, Cross L, Philbin J, Kirstein M. Medication abortion now accounts for more than half of all US abortions. February 24, 2022. Available at: https://www.guttmacher.org/article/2022/02/medication-abortion-now-accounts-more-half-all-us-abortions. Accessed March 1, 2022.
2. Grossman D, White K, Harris L, et al. Continuing pregnancy after mifepristone and "reversal" of first-trimester medical abortion: a systematic review. *Contraception*. 2015;92(3):206–211. https://doi.org/10.1016/j.contraception.2015.06.001
3. Delgado G, Davenport ML. Progesterone use to reverse the effects of mifepristone. *Ann Pharmacother*. 2012;46(12):e36. https://doi.org/10.1345/aph.1R252
4. Garratt D, Turner JV. Progesterone for preventing pregnancy termination after initiation of medical abortion with mifepristone [erratum in *Eur J Contracept Reprod Health Care*. 2017;22(6):I]. *Eur J Contracept Reprod Health Care*. 2017;22(6):472–475. https://doi.org/10.1080/13625187.2017.1412424
5. Delgado G, Condly SJ, Davenport M, et al. A case series detailing the successful reversal of the effects of mifepristone using progesterone. *Issues Law Med*. 2018;33(1):21–31.
6. Creinin MD, Hou MY, Dalton L, Steward R, Chen MJ. Mifepristone antagonization with progesterone to prevent medical abortion: a randomized controlled trial. *Obstet Gynecol*. 2020;135(1):158–165. https://doi.org/10.1097/AOG.0000000000003620
7. American College of Obstetrics and Gynecology. Facts are important: medication abortion "reversal" is not supported by science. Available at: https://www.acog.org/advocacy/facts-are-important/medication-abortion-reversal-is-not-supported-by-science. Accessed March 15, 2020.

8. Grossman D, White K. Abortion "reversal"—legislating without evidence. *N Engl J Med.* 2018;379(16):1491–1493. https://doi.org/10.1056/NEJMp1805927
9. Bhatti KZ, Nguyen AT, Stuart GS. Medical abortion reversal: science and politics meet. *Am J Obstet Gynecol.* 2018;218(3):315.e1–315.e6. https://doi.org/10.1016/j.ajog.2017.11.555
10. McLemore M. Explained: so-called "abortion reversal." Innovating Education in Reproductive Health, UCSF Bixby Center for Global Reproductive Health. 2018. Available at: https://innovating-education.org/2018/03/explained-so-called-abortion-reversal. Accessed April 15, 2022.
11. Salehijam M. The value of systematic content analysis in legal research. *Tilburg Law Review.* 2018;23:34–42. https://doi.org/10.5334/tilr.5
12. The Policy Surveillance Program. Medication abortion requirements. Available at: http://lawatlas.org/datasets/medication-abortion-requirements. Accessed January 15, 2022.
13. Ark Code Ann §20-16-1703 (2015).
14. W Va Code §16-2I-2 (2021).
15. Tenn Code Ann §39-15-218 (2020).
16. Ind Code Ann §16-34-2-1 (2021).
17. La Rev Stat §40:1061.11.1 (2021).
18. Ariz Rev Stat §36-2153 (2016).
19. Ky Rev Stat §311.725 (2019).
20. Utah Code Ann §76-7-305 (2018).
21. 63 Okla Stat §1-756 (2019).
22. Neb Rev Stat § 28-327 (2019).
23. Mont Code Ann 50-20-707 (2021).
24. Redd SK, Hall KS, Aswani MS, Sen B, Wingate M, Rice WS. Variation in restrictive abortion policies and adverse birth outcomes in the United States from 2005 to 2015. *Womens Health Issues.* 2022;32(2):103–113. https://doi.org/10.1016/j.whi.2021.10.006
25. Jones RK, Jerman J. Abortion incidence and service availability in the United States, 2014. *Perspect Sex Reprod Health.* 2017;49(1):17–27. https://doi.org/10.1363/psrh.12015
26. Cairney P, Oliver K. Evidence-based policymaking is not like evidence-based medicine, so how far should you go to bridge the divide between evidence and policy? *Health Res Policy Syst.* 2017;15(1):35. https://doi.org/10.1186/s12961-017-0192-x
27. Kreitzer RJ. Politics and morality in state abortion policy. *State Polit Policy Q.* 2015;15(1):41–66. https://doi.org/10.1177/1532440014561868
28. Hartig H. About six-in-ten Americans say abortion should be legal in all or most cases. Pew Research Center. 2022. Available at: https://www.pewresearch.org/fact-tank/2022/06/13/about-six-in-ten-americans-say-abortion-should-be-legal-in-all-or-most-cases-2. Accessed August 15, 2022.
29. Medoff MH, Dennis C. TRAP abortion laws and partisan political party control of state government. *Am J Econ Sociol.* 2011;70(4):951–973. https://doi.org/10.1111/j.1536-7150.2011.00794.x
30. Pacheco J. Measuring and evaluating changes in state opinion across eight issues. *Am Polit Res.* 2014;42(6):986–1009. https://doi.org/10.1177/1532673X14524819
31. Center for Reproductive Rights. After Roe fell: abortion laws by state. Available at: https://reproductiverights.org/maps/abortion-laws-by-state. Accessed August 1, 2022.
32. Kumar A, Hessini L, Mitchell EM. Conceptualising abortion stigma. *Cult Health Sex.* 2009;11(6):625–639. https://doi.org/10.1080/13691050902842741
33. Foster DG, Gould H, Taylor J, Weitz TA. Attitudes and decision making among women seeking abortions at one US clinic. *Perspect Sex Reprod Health.* 2012;44(2):117–124. https://doi.org/10.1363/4411712
34. Ralph LJ, Foster DG, Kimport K, Turok D, Roberts SCM. Measuring decisional certainty among women seeking abortion. *Contraception.* 2017;95(3):269–278. https://doi.org/10.1016/j.contraception.2016.09.008
35. Jovel I, Cartwright AF, Ralph L, Upadhyay UD. Abortion waiting periods and decision certainty among people searching online for abortion care. *Obstet Gynecol.* 2021;137(4):597–605. https://doi.org/10.1097/AOG.0000000000004313
36. Turan JM, Budhwani H. Restrictive abortion laws exacerbate stigma, resulting in harm to patients and providers. *Am J Public Health.* 2021;111(1):37–39. https://doi.org/10.2105/AJPH.2020.305998
37. Biggs MA, Brown K, Foster DG. Perceived abortion stigma and psychological well-being over five years after receiving or being denied an abortion. *PLoS One.* 2020;15(1):e0226417. https://doi.org/10.1371/journal.pone.0226417
38. Swartzendruber A, English A, Greenberg KB, et al. Crisis pregnancy centers in the United States: lack of adherence to medical and ethical practice standards; a joint position statement of the Society for Adolescent Health and Medicine and the North American Society for Pediatric and Adolescent Gynecology. *J Pediatr Adolesc Gynecol.* 2019;32(6):563–566. https://doi.org/10.1016/j.jpag.2019.10.008
39. Abortion Pill Rescue Network. Abortion pill reversal. Available at: https://abortionpillreversal.com. Accessed March 15, 2022.
40. Harvard T.H. Chan School of Public Health. The public's perspective on the United States public health system. Robert Wood Johnson Foundation/Harvard School of Public Health. May 13, 2021. Available at: https://www.rwjf.org/en/library/research/2021/05/the-publics-perspective-on-the-united-states-public-health-system.html. Accessed August 20, 2022.
41. Redd SK, Rice WS, Aswani MS, et al. Racial/ethnic and educational inequities in restrictive abortion policy variation and adverse birth outcomes in the United States. *BMC Health Serv Res.* 2021;21(1):1139. https://doi.org/10.1186/s12913-021-07165-x
42. Sudhinaraset M, Vilda D, Gipson JD, Bornstein M, Wallace ME. Women's reproductive rights policies and adverse birth outcomes: a state-level analysis to assess the role of race and nativity status. *Am J Prev Med.* 2020;59(6):787–795. https://doi.org/10.1016/j.amepre.2020.07.025
43. Mosley EA, Redd SK, Hartwig SA, et al. Racial and ethnic abortion disparities following Georgia's 22-week gestational age limit. *Womens Health Issues.* 2022;32(1):9–19. https://doi.org/10.1016/j.whi.2021.09.005
44. Rice WS, Labgold K, Peterson QT, Higdon M, Njoku O. Sociodemographic and service use characteristics of abortion fund cases from six states in the US Southeast. *Int J Environ Res Public Health.* 2021;18(7):3813. https://doi.org/10.3390/ijerph18073813
45. Guttmacher Institute. Evidence you can use: mandatory counseling for abortion. January 22, 2020. Available at: https://www.guttmacher.org/evidence-you-can-use/mandatory-counseling-abortion. Accessed August 20, 2022.
46. Weinberger SE, Lawrence HC 3rd, Henley DE, Alden ER, Hoyt DB. Legislative interference with the patient–physician relationship. *N Engl J Med.* 2012;367(16):1557–1559. https://doi.org/10.1056/NEJMsb1209858
47. Mercier RJ, Buchbinder M, Bryant A, Britton L. The experiences and adaptations of abortion providers practicing under a new TRAP law: a qualitative study. *Contraception.* 2015;91(6):507–512. https://doi.org/10.1016/j.contraception.2015.03.003

Insurance-Based Discrimination Reports and Access to Care Among Nonelderly US Adults, 2011–2019

Kathleen Thiede Call, PhD, Giovann Alarcon-Espinoza, PhD, MPP, Natalie Schwer Mac Arthur, PhD, MAc, and Rhonda Jones-Webb, DrPH

See also Spencer and Chen, p. 141.

Objectives. To report insurance-based discrimination rates for nonelderly adults with private, public, or no insurance between 2011 and 2019, a period marked by passage and implementation of the Affordable Care Act (ACA) and threats to it.

Methods. We used 2011–2019 data from the biennial Minnesota Health Access Survey. Each year, about 4000 adults aged 18 to 64 years report experiences with insurance-based discrimination. Using logistic regressions, we examined associations between insurance-based discrimination and (1) sociodemographic factors and (2) indicators of access.

Results. Insurance-based discrimination was stable over time and consistently related to insurance type: approximately 4% for adults with private insurance compared with adults with public insurance (21%) and no insurance (27%). Insurance-based discrimination persistently interfered with confidence in getting needed care and forgoing care.

Conclusions. Policy changes from 2011 to 2019 affected access to health insurance, but high rates of insurance-based discrimination among adults with public insurance or no insurance were impervious to such changes.

Public Health Implications. Stable rates of insurance-based discrimination during a time of increased access to health insurance via the ACA suggest deeper structural roots of health care inequities. We recommend several policy and system solutions. (*Am J Public Health.* 2023;113(2):213–223. https://doi.org/10.2105/AJPH.2022.307126)

AJPH February 2023, Vol 113, No. 2

Health insurance is not a universal right in the United States. Consequently, people lacking health insurance face greater barriers to accessing primary care and timely sick care.[1,2] Furthermore, access to health insurance in the United States is based on an individual's or group's resources. Private insurance is available to some through employment or their financial ability to pay; public insurance is available to some with low incomes or who meet categorical eligibility (e.g., elderly, disabled, children), whereas others remain uninsured, citing inability to afford coverage and ineligibility for existing coverage as top barriers.[1] Health insurance systems that are based on individual resources can lead to inequities—such as insurance-based discrimination—and perpetuate the notion that some people are more deserving of receiving care than others.

Insurance-based discrimination refers to unfair treatment that patients receive from health care providers because of the type of insurance they have (or because they do not have insurance). As is true of all forms of discrimination, insurance-based discrimination manifests at multiple levels: individual (e.g., internalized shame for needing assistance), interpersonal (e.g., treated with disrespect, told they are wasting taxpayer money),[3] and institutional (e.g., policies and practices in organizations that provide differential access to services).[4] Insurance-based discrimination at the interpersonal level is rooted and reinforced in policies like lower physician compensation for Medicaid services than for Medicare and private insurance, which results in differential treatment, such as instructions to schedulers to prioritize private over public pay patients, long wait times, separation of public and private pay patients in academic medical center clinics, and narrow networks where providers do not accept new Medicaid patients.[5–10]

Past research consistently shows dramatically higher rates of insurance-based discrimination among people with public rather than private insurance.[3,11–15] Past research also consistently demonstrates that reports of insurance-based discrimination are tied to delayed and forgone care,[3,12,13] lack of confidence in getting needed care,[12] reports of poor-quality care,[7] and receipt of suboptimal care.[14] Experiences of discrimination are also associated with using more costly emergency department services instead of primary care.[3]

The 2010 passage of the Affordable Care Act (ACA) represents one of several federal efforts to address inequities in access to health insurance, health care, and, possibly, insurance-based discrimination. Beginning in 2014, states that expanded Medicaid received a 100% federal match to encourage covering a broader group of people with low incomes. To ensure an adequate supply of providers, the ACA also mandated a 2-year increase in physician payment rates for Medicaid to the level of Medicare,[5] yet this was not enough to stem the financial preference for private over public patients.[6] The individual mandate (i.e., the requirement to have insurance or face a penalty) held promise for reducing stigma attached to insurance available through government interventions because public insurance was the only affordable option for some people to meet this requirement.[16] However, in 2017, the new presidential administration set this penalty at zero, marking the first challenge to the ACA. Other efforts to dismantle the ACA followed, along with renewed efforts to tie notions of deservedness to public insurance, such as state attempts to link work requirements to Medicaid.[17]

By all measures, the ACA was successful in expanding insurance coverage and lowering uninsured rates, mostly through large gains in Medicaid enrollment.[1] Evidence of gains in access and quality of care for adults with public versus private insurance is mixed. Some studies reported similar access to outpatient care, affordability, and quality ratings for adults with both forms of insurance.[2] Other studies found that adults with private insurance fared better in terms of stability of coverage, affordability, having a personal physician, and obtaining specialist and dental care.[2,18,19] However, adults with private insurance reported less financial protection and were more likely to report medical debt than Medicaid beneficiaries.[2,18]

The controversial nature of the ACA's passage, its incremental implementation, and repeated efforts to repeal it begs the question of whether ongoing public and policy debates surrounding this legislation have influenced insurance-based discrimination and, in turn, access to health care among those most vulnerable. Extending coverage to a broader group of people may not eliminate experiences of insurance-based discrimination given long-standing negative views of public insurance in health care and society. This assumption is supported by dueling terms surrounding the ACA—the "woodwork" and "welcome mat" effects—which indicate polarized opinions in public and policy circles. The former term insinuates that people previously eligible now "crawl out of the woodwork" to enroll in Medicaid, as opposed to "welcoming" enrollment with the latter.[20] This important question has not been addressed in the research on insurance-based discrimination. Past research has provided single-year snapshots of the presence and impact of insurance-based discrimination on access to health care, yet almost all studies precede either ACA passage[3,11,14,15,21–23] or full implementation.[12,24] The exception is the study by Skopec and Long, who use data from 2016, which is after full implementation but before the change of administration and formal efforts to repeal.[13] This article addresses important gaps in current research on insurance-based discrimination, health care access, and the ACA.

The specific objectives of this article are to (1) examine experiences of insurance-based discrimination in Minnesota from 2011 to 2019, (2) describe the correlates of insurance-based discrimination, and (3) investigate the association between insurance-based discrimination and health care access. Our study covers the early years of ACA implementation (which were marked by challenges to Medicaid expansion[17]), through full implementation (marked by state variation in Medicaid expansion and launch of Marketplace plans), through a change of administration (marked by efforts to dismantle the ACA and create obstacles to Medicaid enrollment), through a subsequent change of administration backing ACA initiatives; the study stops, however, before the onset of the COVID-19 pandemic. Understanding these events and their impact on public policy and opinion is an important step in grasping how broader forces operate in shaping insurance-based discrimination in our health care system, how insurance-based discrimination relates to health care access over time, and what can be done to reduce insurance-based discrimination. Results may be informative to health care institutions and policymakers seeking effective multilevel and multicomponent strategies to reduce inequities in health care delivery.

METHODS

Data were from the Minnesota Health Access Survey (MNHA), a biennial survey representative of the noninstitutionalized population in Minnesota. The MNHA undersamples older adults and oversamples rural populations and areas with concentrations of individuals who identify as racial or ethnic minority, and those with lower incomes. The MNHA collects information about sociodemographic characteristics, health insurance coverage, and access to care for a randomly selected household member. We used data from 2011, 2013, 2015, 2017, and 2019. However, 2 changes in the survey design in 2019 limit comparability with previous years. First, the 2019 MNHA added an address-based sample frame to the standard dual random digit dialing frame used in previous years. Second, the address-based sample frame collected data primarily through a computer-assisted Web interview program. This change in survey administration, from interacting directly with an interviewer to answering the questions via self-guided Web site, could affect respondents' reports of discrimination in 2019.

Sample

We restricted the population to nonelderly adults aged 18–64 years because of the high uptake of Medicare among adults aged older than 64 years and enduring differences in narratives of deservedness between Medicare and Medicaid.[7] We also excluded proxy reports, such as responding for a child or a spouse. Limiting the analysis to adults responding for themselves about insurance and experiences of discrimination provides a more conscientious examination of the association between insurance-based discrimination and insurance type (Table 1).

Consistent with national trends, response rates decreased over time from 44% (2011) to 22% (2019).[25] Because of the 2019 change in sampling strategy, we retroactively implemented the updated weighting approach to all previous years of data. We weighted data to adjust for nonresponse bias and to reflect the general population in Minnesota.[26]

Measures

The MNHA asks, "How often do health care providers treat you unfairly because of the type of health insurance you have?" or "because you don't have health insurance?" We coded someone as experiencing insurance-based discrimination if they reported that health care providers always, usually, or sometimes (vs never) treated them unfairly because of their health insurance (or lack thereof). The survey also includes a measure of race-based discrimination ("How often do health care providers treat you unfairly because of your race, ethnicity, or nationality?").

We measured insurance type by providing a list of responses that we recoded as private insurance (i.e., employer-sponsored, self-purchased, and, starting in 2015, MNsure [Minnesota's Marketplace plan]) or public insurance (i.e., Medicare, Medicaid, MinnesotaCare). We coded respondents reporting both private and public insurance as having public because of our research focus on public insurance. Consistent with federal surveys, we classified adults responding no to all sources (or who reported only Indian Health Services) as uninsured.

We examined 3 indicators of access: (1) usual source of care (excluding emergency departments), (2) confidence in getting care when needed (very or somewhat confident vs a little or not at all confident), and (3) reports of forgone care due to cost in the last 12 months (prescribed medications, dental care, routine care, specialist care, and mental or behavioral care).

The survey included measures tied to societal opportunities, power, and resources such as gender, age, race/ethnicity, nativity, family income, education, marital status, employment status, self-reported health status, and place of residency (rural or urban).

Analyses

We examined reports of insurance-based discrimination among nonelderly adults from 2011 to 2019. We used the *t*-test to assess differences in rates over time ($P < .05$) and logistic regressions to assess associations between (1) insurance-based discrimination and sociodemographic factors and (2) insurance-based discrimination and health care access. Given widespread evidence of race-based discrimination in health care, our sensitivity analysis also adjusted for race-based discrimination.[17,22] We followed current recommendations to select reference groups in our analysis.[27] We clustered regressions to estimate robust standard errors and report adjusted odds ratios (AORs).

TABLE 1— Sociodemographic Characteristics, Health Status, and Health Care Access by Year Among Adults Aged 18–64 Years: Minnesota, 2011–2019

	2011, No. or %	2013, No. or %	2015, No. or %	2017, No. or %	2019, No. or %
Unweighted sample size	4024	4157	3934	4635	4365
Type of health insurance, %					
Private	71.1	71.6	73.3	69.6*	70.8
Public	17.4	17.7	23.1*	22.8	22.1
Uninsured	11.5	10.7	3.6*	7.7*	7.1
Gender, %					
Male	43.3	46.8	47.6	46.0	41.0*
Female	56.7	53.2	52.4	54.0	59.0*
Race and ethnicity, %					
Hispanic	4.3	4.6	4.9	4.9	5.3
White	84.4	83.2	82.2	80.8	81.3
Black	4.5	5.4	5.7	6.0	5.8
Asian	4.7	5.3	5.5	5.4	5.8
American Indian	1.4	1.4	1.5	2.1	1.5
Other	—[a]	—[a]	—[a]	0.8*	—[a]
Country of birth, %					
Not US-born	9.9	11.1	12.2	12.1	11.6
US-born	90.1	88.9	87.8	87.9	88.5
Age, y, %					
18–25	14.5	17.1	14.4	15.0	14.8
26–34	20.1	18.7	21.6	20.8	21.2
35–54	45.9	43.6	42.7	42.3	41.6
55–64	19.5	20.7	21.3	21.9	22.4
Family income, % of FPG					
0–138	15.4	15.9	16.0	13.8	14.7
139–250	16.3	15.5	15.5	16.6	13.7
251–400	24.3	24.7	24.7	20.3*	20.2
> 400	44.0	43.9	43.8	49.4*	51.4
Education, %					
No high school diploma	6.0	7.1	6.5	7.3	4.8*
High school diploma or GED	25.6	25.6	22.9	23.8	20.2
Some college	35.2	35.3	35.3	35.3	35.3
Bachelor's degree	23.4	22.7	24.2	23.6	26.9*
Postgraduate	9.9	9.3	11.2	10.1	12.8*
Marital status, %					
Not married	37.8	40.5	39.1	43.3*	39.2*
Married	62.2	59.5	61.0	56.7*	60.8*
Employment status, %					
Employed	77.4	81.0	82.1	82.9	81.6
Not employed	22.7	19.0	17.9	17.1	18.4
Place of residence, %					
Urban	73.3	73.3	74.7	73.0	73.6
Rural	26.7	26.7	25.3	27.1	26.4
Health status, %					
Excellent, very good, or good	90.6	87.8*	88.5	86.5	86.8

Continued

TABLE 1— Continued

	2011, No. or %	2013, No. or %	2015, No. or %	2017, No. or %	2019, No. or %
Fair or poor	9.4	12.2*	11.5	13.5	13.2
Usual source of care (other than emergency department), %					
Had a usual source of care	81.9	80.1	82.3	80.5	81.3
Lacked a usual source of care	18.1	20.0	17.7	19.5	18.7
Confidence in getting needed care, %					
Had confidence	88.1	88.9	91.2	87.4*	88.4
Lacked confidence	11.9	11.1	8.8	12.7*	11.6
Any forgone care due to cost in past year, %[b]					
Did not forgo care	65.9	75.1*	74.9	72.1	63.8*
Forgone care	34.1	24.9*	25.1	27.9	36.2*

Note. FPG = federal poverty guidelines (https://aspe.hhs.gov/topics/poverty-economic-mobility/poverty-guidelines).
Source. Minnesota Health Access Survey. Data were weighted to represent the state's population.

[a]Suppressed, relative standard error > 30.
[b]Any reports of forgone care due to cost including prescribed medications, dental care, routine care, and specialist care in the last 12 months; beginning in 2013, mental or behavioral care was added.
*Indicates a statistically significant change with respect to the previous year ($P < .05$).

RESULTS

Table 1 describes the nonelderly adult sample each year. Full implementation of the ACA resulted in a significant decrease in the uninsured rate between 2013 and 2015 (10.7% to 3.6%, respectively) and a corresponding increase in public insurance enrollment (17.7% to 23.1%). Most adults were covered by private insurance; however, the decrease in private insurance for adults between 2015 and 2017 (73.3% to 69.6%) corresponded with an increase in uninsurance (3.6% to 7.7%).

On average, approximately 10% of nonelderly adults reported insurance-based discrimination (Figure 1), although this increased from 7.7% in 2015 to 11.0% in 2017, the same year that the uninsured rate doubled and private insurance dropped significantly (Table 1). Reports of insurance-based discrimination by type of insurance were stable between 2011 and 2019, ranging from 24.7% to 28.1% for uninsured adults and 18.4% to 24.0% for publicly insured adults, compared with 3.0% to 5.4% for adults with private insurance. In terms of our access measures, fewer than 20% of adults reported lacking a usual source of care, fewer than 13% reported lacking confidence in receiving needed care, and fewer than 37% reported forgone care over the study period.

Correlates of Insurance-Based Discrimination

Three sociodemographic characteristics were consistently associated with insurance-based discrimination over the period of analysis: type of health insurance, income, and health status (Table 2). Being uninsured showed a consistent association with insurance-based discrimination in all years (AORs ranged from 3.63 to 9.40). Having public coverage was associated with insurance-based discrimination in all years except 2017.

Minnesotan adults with greater family income relative to the federal poverty guidelines (https://aspe.hhs.gov/topics/poverty-economic-mobility/poverty-guidelines) had consistently lower odds of experiencing insurance-based discrimination compared with families with income below 139% of the federal poverty guidelines. Adults reporting "fair" or "poor" health status had about double the odds of reporting insurance-based discrimination as those with better self-reported health.

We tested the robustness of our results by adding race-based discrimination to our model. Reports of race-based and insurance-based discrimination were highly associated. However, even when we adjusted for race-based discrimination, insurance-based discrimination remained highly associated with health insurance, income, and health status (Appendix A, available as a supplement to the online version of this article at http://www.ajph.org).

Discrimination and Access to Health Care

We found that people who experienced insurance-based discrimination were

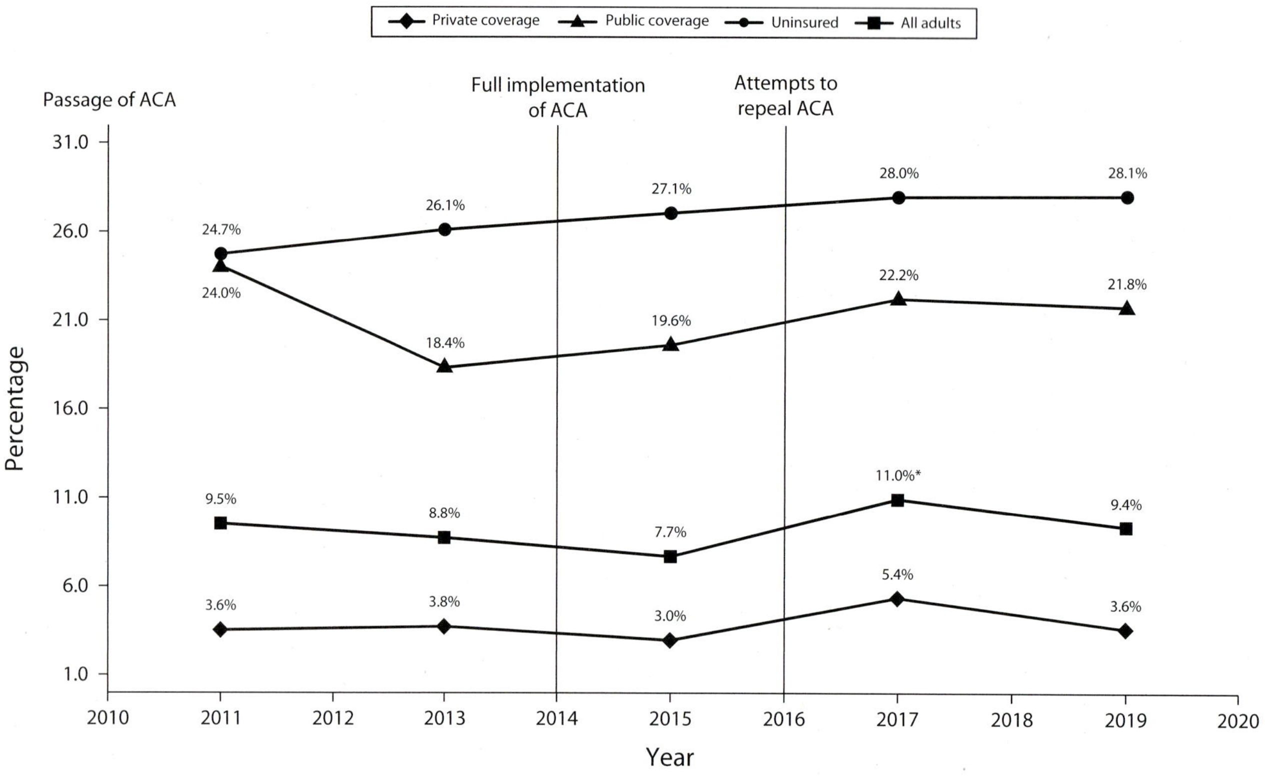

FIGURE 1— Reports of Insurance-Based Discrimination Among Nonelderly Adults and by Type of Health Insurance Among Adults (Aged 18–64 Years): Minnesota, 2011–2019

Note. ACA = Affordable Care Act.
Source. Minnesota Health Access Survey. Data were weighted to represent the state's population.
*Indicates a statistically significant change with respect to the previous year ($P < .05$).

more likely to report forgoing care because of costs in all 5 years observed (AORs ranged from 2.39 to 4.64; Table 3 and online Appendix B). Insurance-based discrimination was associated with increased odds of lacking confidence in getting needed care in 4 of 5 years (AORs ranged from 3.03 to 9.16). Having a usual source of care was not consistently associated with insurance-based discrimination. The results were robust in models including race-based discrimination (online Appendix C).

DISCUSSION

Although more Minnesota adults gained public coverage and fewer adults were uninsured following ACA implementation, reports of insurance-based discrimination by type of insurance remained remarkably stable between 2011 and 2019. Compared with adults with private insurance (4% on average), insurance-based discrimination was 5 or 6 times higher for adults with public insurance (21% on average) and about 7 times higher for adults with no insurance (27% on average). Consistent with past research, there was little association between insurance-based discrimination and having a usual source of care.[3] However, insurance-based discrimination persistently interfered with confidence in getting needed care and reports of forgoing care. These access barriers for adults reporting insurance-based discrimination hold even when we account for reports of race-based discrimination, which is important given historical and ongoing race-based discrimination in the United States.[17,22] This suggests that insurance-based and race-based discrimination are both important to address in creating equitable access to health care. Future analysis will examine these intersecting forces of discrimination more deeply.

To our knowledge, this study is the first to examine rates of insurance-based discrimination over time following passage and full implementation of the ACA. The association between insurance-based discrimination and income was strong even when we controlled for type of health insurance (Table 2). This direct association between income and insurance-based discrimination suggests that adults with lower incomes are more

TABLE 2— Association Between Insurance-Based Discrimination and Insurance Type, Participant Characteristics, and Health Status Among Adults Aged 18–64 Years: Minnesota, 2011–2019

	2011, AOR (95% CI)	2013,[a] AOR (95% CI)	2015, AOR (95% CI)	2017, AOR (95% CI)	2019, AOR (95% CI)
Type of health insurance (Ref: private)					
Public	5.00 (3.87, 6.46)	2.69 (1.44, 5.04)	3.96 (2.83, 5.54)	1.96 (0.98, 3.92)	3.67 (2.21, 6.08)
Uninsured	5.90 (3.39, 10.25)	5.07 (2.57, 9.99)	9.40 (3.98, 22.19)	3.63 (1.89, 6.98)	5.85 (2.88, 11.91)
Female (Ref: male)	1.42 (1.01, 1.99)	0.86 (0.61, 1.21)	1.48 (1.15, 1.90)	1.27 (0.79, 2.05)	1.30 (0.75, 2.26)
Race and ethnicity (Ref: Hispanic)					
White	0.73 (0.26, 2.01)	3.09 (0.43, 22.13)	5.43 (2.05, 14.40)	0.97 (0.31, 3.05)	0.69 (0.31, 1.55)
Black	1.59 (0.88, 2.85)	6.02 (0.67, 53.86)	6.35 (3.54, 11.40)	0.74 (0.27, 2.03)	1.47 (0.23, 9.52)
Asian	1.43 (0.33, 6.21)	2.85 (0.49, 16.66)	7.23 (2.24, 23.36)	0.61 (0.25, 1.51)	0.40 (0.22, 0.72)
American Indian	1.37 (0.44, 4.29)	4.72 (0.74, 30.02)	6.77 (1.10, 41.58)	2.51 (0.65, 9.68)	1.43 (0.38, 5.36)
Other	0.88 (0.20, 3.91)	. . .	2.91 (0.99, 8.59)	2.17 (0.64, 7.33)	4.59 (2.40, 8.77)
US-born (Ref: not US-born)	1.68 (1.12, 2.53)	0.59 (0.20, 1.75)	0.25 (0.12, 0.51)	0.71 (0.22, 2.35)	0.85 (0.54, 1.34)
Age, y (Ref: 18–25)					
26–34	1.38 (0.70, 2.72)	2.97 (0.82, 10.77)	1.03 (0.54, 1.95)	1.37 (0.56, 3.36)	0.77 (0.40, 1.51)
35–54	1.09 (0.35, 3.42)	1.46 (0.44, 4.85)	0.93 (0.45, 1.92)	2.18 (0.88, 5.41)	0.94 (0.48, 1.82)
55–64	0.75 (0.34, 1.67)	0.85 (0.22, 3.21)	0.89 (0.43, 1.83)	1.42 (0.71, 2.81)	0.87 (0.55, 1.37)
Family income, % of FPG (Ref: 0–138)					
139–250	1.33 (0.60, 2.91)	0.88 (0.51, 1.49)	0.75 (0.50, 1.12)	0.98 (0.51, 1.87)	0.95 (0.65, 1.37)
251–400	1.04 (0.42, 2.58)	0.37 (0.15, 0.88)	0.37 (0.21, 0.63)	0.58 (0.26, 1.30)	0.34 (0.20, 0.56)
> 400	0.89 (0.55, 1.45)	0.32 (0.11, 0.90)	0.21 (0.12, 0.35)	0.36 (0.17, 0.76)	0.30 (0.18, 0.48)
Education (Ref: no high school diploma)					
High school diploma	0.66 (0.21, 2.10)	3.08 (0.91, 10.38)	0.87 (0.44, 1.72)	0.61 (0.36, 1.05)	1.12 (0.34, 3.66)
Some college	0.70 (0.20, 2.45)	2.94 (1.35, 6.39)	1.40 (0.77, 2.54)	0.59 (0.33, 1.04)	2.82 (0.80, 9.96)
Bachelor's degree	0.65 (0.17, 2.52)	2.17 (0.75, 6.31)	0.75 (0.40, 1.40)	0.45 (0.25, 0.80)	2.27 (0.56, 9.29)
Postgraduate studies	0.51 (0.07, 3.68)	1.94 (0.39, 9.64)	0.96 (0.50, 1.85)	0.26 (0.10, 0.67)	1.64 (0.29, 9.28)
Married (Ref: not married)	0.60 (0.34, 1.05)	0.82 (0.50, 1.34)	1.01 (0.71, 1.45)	0.52 (0.27, 1.01)	0.53 (0.35, 0.81)
Employed (Ref: not employed)	1.06 (0.81, 1.39)	1.01 (0.59, 1.75)	0.85 (0.46, 1.56)	1.23 (0.75, 2.00)	0.59 (0.42, 0.83)
Rural (Ref: urban)	0.92 (0.46, 1.83)	1.20 (0.56, 2.61)	1.10 (0.58, 2.08)	1.20 (0.72, 2.03)	0.80 (0.48, 1.34)
Fair/poor health status (Ref: excellent, very good, or good)	2.88 (1.85, 4.49)	2.36 (1.64, 3.40)	2.45 (1.38, 4.33)	1.44 (0.94, 2.20)	1.80 (0.91, 3.57)
Sample size	3958	4022	3763	4467	4245

Note. AOR = adjusted odds ratio; CI = confidence interval; FPG = federal poverty guidelines (https://aspe.hhs.gov/topics/poverty-economic-mobility/poverty-guidelines).
Source. Minnesota Health Access Survey. Data were weighted to represent the state's population.

[a]In 2013, results for other race were suppressed because of small sample size, which produced a lack of convergence in the model.

likely to experience discrimination regardless of the type of insurance they have.

Limitations

Our study provides important information about persistent reports of insurance-based discrimination and its negative association with access to care, but there are limitations. First, the data are repeat cross-sections measuring insurance type and access experiences at the time of the survey and forgone care in the past 12 months, which unfortunately impeded our ability to establish causal associations. Second, we use data from 1 state—Minnesota, a state with historically high rates of private insurance, low uninsured rates, generous public program eligibility prior to the ACA, and early participation in Medicaid expansion. Nevertheless, our results are consistent

TABLE 3— Association Between 3 Access Measures and Insurance-Based Discrimination Among Adults Aged 18–64 Years: Minnesota, 2011–2019

	2011, AOR (95% CI)	2013, AOR (95% CI)	2015, AOR (95% CI)	2017, AOR (95% CI)	2019, AOR (95% CI)
Lack of usual source of care	2.07 (1.31, 3.27)	1.69 (0.86, 3.33)	1.26 (0.80, 1.97)	1.38 (0.92, 2.09)	0.77 (0.46, 1.31)
Lack of confidence in getting needed care	3.03 (1.92, 4.76)	1.74 (0.68, 4.43)	5.28 (2.95, 9.47)	4.77 (2.45, 9.31)	9.16 (5.99, 13.99)
Forgone care due to cost in past year[a]	2.39 (1.53, 3.74)	4.64 (2.87, 7.51)	4.24 (2.91, 6.16)	2.48 (1.45, 4.22)	3.26 (2.55, 4.17)

Note. AOR = adjusted odds ratio; CI = confidence interval. All models were adjusted for health insurance, gender, race/ethnicity, nativity, age, poverty, education, marital status, employment status, place of residence, and health status.
Source. Minnesota Health Access Survey. Data were weighted to represent the state's population.

[a]Any reports of forgone care due to cost, including prescribed medications, dental care, routine care, and specialist care in the last 12 months; beginning in 2013, mental or behavioral care was added.

with past single-year studies in other states[3,14,15,23] and at the national level.[13,22,24] Third, our single-item measure of insurance-based discrimination is straightforward and easy to administer, yet it admittedly lacks a specific time reference. Thus, people who recently changed coverage (e.g., public to private) may be reporting their experiences with providers based on their prior insurance. However, the associations we report between insurance-based discrimination and type of insurance are consistent with other studies using measures with no time referent,[3,14,21,22] studies that reference a specific hospitalization,[24] and studies that reference the past 6 months[23] or the past 12 months.[13,15]

Fourth, we cannot confidently identify nonelderly people who have Medicaid and Medicare (because of health challenges and disability); their experience with insurance-based discrimination is likely to be more nuanced than that of someone with only Medicaid and in relatively better health. Finally, our measure refers to "health care providers" generally rather than specific roles or provider types (staff, nurse, physician, etc.). This is both consistent with all insurance-based discrimination measures we reviewed and pragmatic, because each clinical encounter involves interactions with a variety of people who shape the experience. For instance, negative stereotypes about uninsured, low-income, and publicly insured patients held by physicians can set the tone for clinic staff.[8]

Public Health Implications

High rates of insurance-based discrimination among nonelderly adults with public insurance and those who lack health insurance were impervious to political and policy shifts between 2011 and 2019, suggesting that this inequity has deeper structural roots. Although insurance-based discrimination is experienced at individual and interpersonal levels, these instances are intertwined with structural and institutional policies such that structural solutions are needed.

Policy solutions. Implementing a single-payer system of coverage that prioritizes our multiracial working class may be a possible solution to addressing insurance-based discrimination. As of 2020, 63% of US adults agreed that "it is the federal government's responsibility to make sure all Americans have health care coverage," with 36% favoring a single national government program.[28] Additionally, beginning in 2016, just over 50% of persons in the United States supported "a national health plan, sometimes called Medicare-for-all, in which all Americans would get their insurance from a single government plan."[29] Although not a panacea, assigning everyone the same insurance removes 1 layer of structural discrimination inherent in a system where people with more resources have private insurance and people with fewer resources have public insurance or no insurance.

Even with a single-payer system, societal perspectives of worth based on income may persist and take the place of insurance-based discrimination. Given the pervasiveness of insurance-based and other forms of discrimination, we also encourage greater structural competency at all levels of government, health care systems, and society. Qualitative research indicates that lower-income patients feel disrespected, ignored, and devalued by health care professionals compared with middle-income patients.[30] Some reported that providers downplayed their health concerns and involved them less in decisions when on public insurance compared with their experience when covered by private insurance.[30] Metzl and Hansen argue for structural competency training for health professionals to overcome the stereotype that people in poverty are more difficult to treat and to instead recognize the complexity of circumstances—social, economic, and political—that make achieving good health extremely challenging for people with low incomes.[31] Shifting blame from people to the structural barriers to power and resources among poor and marginalized people holds promise for reducing insurance-based discrimination.

A second policy solution focuses on altering reimbursement rates for public insurance programs. In the current health care system, it is rational for providers to treat patients with private insurance better than patients with public insurance, whether intentional or not; they are literally paid to do so. States are already exploring ways to structure Medicaid payments and incentives for providers and managed care organizations to define and meet health equity priorities, and some are engaging the community in setting these goals.[32] However, it is critical to monitor whether financing changes translates into improved patient experiences or into greater burden for providers, which, in turn, may increase reports of unfair treatment by Medicaid enrollees. Furthermore, changing incentives is not the same as altogether removing the profit motive from health care.

Institutional and systems solutions. Improved monitoring of insurance-based discrimination in health care is both necessary and possible, as evidenced by inclusion in the supplemental Cultural Competence Item Set of the Consumer Assessment of Healthcare Providers & Systems, a national survey of patients' experiences with health care administered by the Agency for Healthcare Research and Quality.[33] We endorse the call for direct measures of discrimination (e.g., insurance-based discrimination, race-based discrimination) rather than only proxy measures (e.g., insurance type, race, ethnicity) in these monitoring efforts.[34] The Centers for Medicare and Medicaid Services could mandate their use and reward systems with low and improved rates of discrimination. The ACA set out to strengthen nondiscrimination policies. Reporting acts of discrimination was initially required; however, notification expectations were relaxed in 2019.[17] Regardless of this revision, few people file complaints.[13] This may be through lack of awareness about reporting requirements, lack of knowledge about how to file a report, or lack of confidence that anything will come of a complaint, among other things. Including discrimination measures in ongoing quality assessments removes the burden of reporting from people experiencing discrimination.

Embedding community health workers (CHWs) in health care teams is a promising systems solution to promoting both trust in health care and comfort in reporting suboptimal care. CHWs are trusted and trained members of the historically marginalized communities they represent and serve; they contribute to reducing health inequities through education and advocacy, thus creating a bridge between providers and their patients, who otherwise have little power and voice.[35] CHWs increase the comfort level of patients with whom they share life experiences, which increases their trust and ability to navigate and use health care services.[35] CHWs potentially increase patients' knowledge of their rights, which may foster the reporting of discriminatory encounters.

Monitoring insurance-based discrimination and enforcing antidiscrimination policies are important because even though we found reports of insurance-based discrimination to be stable over time, exposure to insurance-based discrimination is growing at the rate of public program enrollment growth. As shown in the current study and past research, insurance-based discrimination consistently results in delayed and forgone care.[3,12,23]

SUMMARY

We examined insurance-based discrimination and access to health care during the creation and implementation of—as well as challenge to—the ACA. We found that during this period, insurance-based discrimination persisted despite increased access to health insurance, especially public health insurance. We suggest several strategies at the policy and institutional levels to ensure a more equitable health care system that all persons in the United States deserve. AJPH

ABOUT THE AUTHORS

Kathleen Thiede Call is with the School of Public Health, Division of Health Policy and Management, and the State Health Access Data Assistance Center (SHADAC), University of Minnesota, Minneapolis. At the time of this writing, Giovann Alarcon-Espinoza was with the School of Public Health, SHADAC, University of Minnesota, Minneapolis. Natalie Schwer Mac Arthur is with the School of Public Health, State Health Access Data Assistance Center, SHADAC, University of Minnesota, Minneapolis. Rhonda Jones-Webb is with the School of Public Health, Division of Epidemiology and Community Health, University of Minnesota, Minneapolis.

CORRESPONDENCE

Correspondence should be sent to Kathleen Thiede Call, 420 Delaware Street SE, MMC 729, University of Minnesota, Minneapolis, MN 55455 (e-mail: callx001@umn.edu). Reprints can be ordered at http://www.ajph.org by clicking the "Reprints" link.

PUBLICATION INFORMATION

Full Citation: Call KT, Alarcon-Espinoza G, Mac Arthur NS, Jones-Webb R. Insurance-based discrimination reports and access to care among nonelderly US adults, 2011–2019. *Am J Public Health*. 2023; 113(2):213–223.

Acceptance Date: September 10, 2022.

DOI: https://doi.org/10.2105/AJPH.2022.307126

CONTRIBUTORS

K. T. Call contributed to the conceptualization and design, data collection, data interpretation, drafting, and critical revision of the article, and approval of the final version. G. Alarcon-Espinoza contributed to the conceptualization and design, data collection, data analysis and interpretation, drafting, and critical revision of the article, and approval of the final version. N. S. Mac Arthur contributed to the data analysis and interpretation, critical revision of the article, and approval of the final version. R. Jones-Webb contributed to the conceptualization and design, drafting and critical revision of the article, and approval of the final version.

ACKNOWLEDGMENTS

This research was supported by the Minnesota Department of Health, Minnesota Department of Human Services, and SHADAC through a grant from the Robert Wood Johnson Foundation.
We appreciate the contributions of Neha Potlapalli and Sydney Bernard, who conducted literature searches to support this research. We are grateful for the magic of SHADAC staff members Andrea Stewart for copyediting and Lindsey Theis for graphics. We thank Kelly McAnnany for her review of an earlier version of the article and many helpful insights. Finally, we are thankful to the talented staff at SSRS for administering the survey and the thousands of Minnesotans over the years who took the time to complete the survey and share their experiences with insurance coverage and access.

Note. The views expressed here do not necessarily reflect the views of our funders or our employers.

CONFLICTS OF INTEREST

The authors declare no conflicts of interests for this article.

HUMAN PARTICIPANT PROTECTION

This study was approved by the University of Minnesota's institutional review board.

REFERENCES

1. Tolbert J, Orgera K, Damico A. Key facts about the uninsured population. Kaiser Family Foundation. November 6, 2020. Available at: https://www.kff.org/uninsured/issue-brief/key-facts-about-the-uninsured-population. Accessed March 30, 2022.
2. Nguyen KH, Sommers BD. Access and quality of care by insurance type for low-income adults before the Affordable Care Act. *Am J Public Health*. 2016;106(8):1409–1415. https://doi.org/10.2105/AJPH.2016.303156
3. Allen H, Wright BJ, Harding K, Broffman L. The role of stigma in access to health care for the poor. *Milbank Q*. 2014;92(2):289–318. https://doi.org/10.1111/1468-0009.12059
4. Jones CP. Levels of racism: a theoretic framework and a gardener's tale. *Am J Public Health*. 2000; 90(8):1212–1215. https://doi.org/10.2105/AJPH.90.8.1212
5. Zuckerman S, Williams AF, Stockley KE. Trends in Medicaid physician fees, 2003–2008. *Health Aff (Millwood)*. 2009;28(3 suppl 1):w510–w519. https://doi.org/10.1377/hlthaff.28.3.w510
6. Olson J. Mayo to give preference to privately insured patients over Medicaid patients. *StarTribune*. March 15, 2017. Available at: https://www.startribune.com/mayo-to-pick-privately-insured-patients-amid-medicaid-pressures/416185134. Accessed November 5, 2022.
7. Martinez-Hume AC, Baker AM, Bell HS, Montemayor I, Elwell K, Hunt LM. "They treat you a different way": public insurance, stigma, and the challenge to quality health care. *Cult Med Psychiatry*. 2017;41(1):161–180. https://doi.org/10.1007/s11013-016-9513-8
8. Tajeu GS, Cherrington AL, Andreae L, Prince C, Holt CL, Halanych JH. "We'll get to you when we get to you": exploring potential contributions of health care staff behaviors to patient perceptions of discrimination and satisfaction. *Am J Public Health*. 2015;105(10):2076–2082. https://doi.org/10.2105/AJPH.2015.302721
9. Bachhuber MA, Tschannerl A, Lechuga C, Anderson M. Racial discrimination in health care settings: does insurance matter? *Am J Public Health*. 2014;104(3):e10–e11. https://doi.org/10.2105/AJPH.2013.301777
10. Hsiang WR, Lukasiewicz A, Gentry M, et al. Medicaid patients have greater difficulty scheduling health care appointments compared with private insurance patients: a meta-analysis. *Inquiry*. 2019;56:1–9. https://doi.org/10.1177/0046958019838118
11. De Marco M, Thorburn S, Zhao W. Perceived discrimination during prenatal care, labor, and delivery: an examination of data from the Oregon Pregnancy Risk Assessment Monitoring System, 1998–1999, 2000, and 2001. *Am J Public Health*. 2008;98(10):1818–1822. https://doi.org/10.2105/AJPH.2007.123687
12. Han X, Call KT, Pintor JK, Alarcon-Espinoza G, Simon AB. Reports of insurance-based discrimination in health care and its association with access to care. *Am J Public Health*. 2015;105(suppl 3): S517–S525. https://doi.org/10.2105/AJPH.2015.302668
13. Skopec L, Long SK. Poor treatment by health care providers and staff is more common among vulnerable populations. Health Reform Monitoring Survey (HRMS) Brief. October 24, 2016. Available at: https://www.urban.org/sites/default/files/publication/105149/hrms-poor-treatment-brief-webpdf.pdf. Accessed April 1, 2022.
14. Thorburn S, De Marco M. Insurance-based discrimination during prenatal care, labor, and delivery: perceptions of Oregon mothers. *Matern Child Health J*. 2010;14(6):875–885. https://doi.org/10.1007/s10995-009-0533-7
15. Trivedi AN, Ayanian JZ. Perceived discrimination and use of preventive health services. *J Gen Intern Med*. 2006;21(6):553–558. https://doi.org/10.1111/j.1525-1497.2006.00413.x
16. Grogan CM, Park SE. The politics of Medicaid: most Americans are connected to the program, support its expansion, and do not view it as stigmatizing. *Milbank Q*. 2017;95(4):749–782. https://doi.org/10.1111/1468-0009.12298
17. Michener J. Race, politics, and the Affordable Care Act. *J Health Polit Policy Law*. 2020;45(4): 547–566. https://doi.org/10.1215/03616878-8255481
18. Wray CM, Khare M, Keyhani S. Access to care, cost of care, and satisfaction with care among adults with private and public health insurance in the US. *JAMA Netw Open*. 2021;4(6):e2110275. https://doi.org/10.1001/jamanetworkopen.2021.10275
19. Chaiyachati KH, Hom JK, Wong C, et al. Access to primary and dental care among adults newly enrolled in Medicaid. *Am J Manag Care*. 2019;25(3): 135–139.
20. Blewett LA. Medicaid expansion: out of the woodwork or onto the welcome mat? State Health Access Data Assistance Center. October 12, 2012. Updated October 25, 2012. Available at: https://www.shadac.org/news/medicaid-expansion-out-woodwork-or-welcome-mat. Accessed March 30, 2022.
21. Allen EM, Call KT, Beebe TJ, McAlpine DD, Johnson PJ. Barriers to care and healthcare utilization among the publicly insured. *Med Care*. 2017; 55(3):207–214. https://doi.org/10.1097/MLR.0000000000000644
22. Lillie-Blanton M, Brodie M, Rowland D, Altman D, McIntosh M. Race, ethnicity, and the health care system: public perceptions and experiences. *Med Care Res Rev*. 2000;57(suppl 1):218–235. https://doi.org/10.1177/1077558700057001S10
23. Weech-Maldonado R, Hall A, Bryant T, Jenkins KA, Elliott MN. The relationship between perceived discrimination and patient experiences with health care. *Med Care*. 2012;50(9 suppl 2): S62–S68. https://doi.org/10.1097/MLR.0b013e31825fb235
24. Attanasio LB, Hardeman RR. Declined care and discrimination during the childbirth hospitalization. *Soc Sci Med*. 2019;232:270–277. https://doi.org/10.1016/j.socscimed.2019.05.008
25. Czajka JL, Beyler A. Declining response rates in federal surveys: trends and implications. Background Paper. Final Report, Vol. 1. Mathematica Policy Research. Updated June 15, 2016. Available at: https://aspe.hhs.gov/sites/default/files/private/pdf/255531/Decliningresponserates.pdf. Accessed March 1, 2021.
26. Call K. 2019 Minnesota Health Access Survey Technical Report: study design and data processing methodology. State Health Access Data Assistance Center. Updated June 30, 2021. Available at: https://www.shadac.org/publications/MNHA-2019-technical-report. Accessed April 7, 2022.
27. Johfre SS, Freese J. Reconsidering the reference category. *Sociol Methodol*. 2021;51(2):253–269. https://doi.org/10.1177/0081175020982632
28. Jones B. Increasing share of Americans favor a single government program to provide health care coverage. Pew Research Center. September 29, 2020. Available at: https://www.pewresearch.

org/fact-tank/2020/09/29/increasing-share-of-americans-favor-a-single-government-program-to-provide-health-care-coverage. Accessed April 2, 2022.

29. Kaiser Family Foundation. Public opinion on single-payer, national health plans, and expanding access to Medicare coverage. October 16, 2020. Available at: https://www.kff.org/slideshow/public-opinion-on-single-payer-national-health-plans-and-expanding-access-to-medicare-coverage. Accessed April 2, 2022.
30. Duke CC, Stanik C. Overcoming lower-income patients' concerns about trust and respect from providers. Health Affairs Forefront. August 11, 2016. Available at: https://www.healthaffairs.org/do/10.1377/forefront.20160811.056138/full. Accessed April 4, 2022.
31. Metzl JM, Hansen H. Structural competency: theorizing a new medical engagement with stigma and inequality. *Soc Sci Med.* 2014;103:126–133. https://doi.org/10.1016/j.socscimed.2013.06.032
32. Akard J. Improving health equity in Medicaid: state policy innovation and research. AcademyHealth: Health Equity Meeting Blog Series. March 2, 2022. Available at: https://academyhealth.org/blog/2022-03/improving-health-equity-medicaid-state-policy-innovation-and-research. Accessed April 1, 2022.
33. Consumer Assessment of Healthcare Providers & Systems. About the CAHPS® Cultural Competence Item Set. CAHPS® Clinician & Group Surveys and Instructions. Document no. 2312. Updated May 1, 2012. Available at: https://theinstitute.umaryland.edu/media/ssw/institute/national-center-documents/samhsa-sponsored-meetings/Consumer-Assessment-for-Healthcare-and-Provider-Systems-(CAHPS)-Cultural-Competence-Data-Set.pdf. Accessed April 7, 2022.
34. Lett E, Asabor E, Beltrán S, Cannon AM, Arah OA. Conceptualizing, contextualizing, and operationalizing race in quantitative health sciences research. *Ann Fam Med.* 2022;20(2):157–163. https://doi.org/10.1370/afm.2792
35. Cosgrove S, Moore-Monroy M, Jenkins C, et al. Community health workers as an integral strategy in the REACH US program to eliminate health inequities. *Health Promot Pract.* 2014;15(6):795–802. https://doi.org/10.1177/1524839914541442

Rural–Urban Disparities in Adverse Maternal Outcomes in the United States, 2016–2019

Katharine A. Harrington, MPH, Natalie A. Cameron, MD, Kasen Culler, MD, William A. Grobman, MD, MBA, and Sadiya S. Khan, MD, MSc

Objectives. To describe differences in maternal admissions to the intensive care unit (ICU) and mortality in rural versus urban areas in the United States.

Methods. We performed a nationwide analysis and calculated age-standardized rates and rate ratios (RRs) of maternal ICU admission and mortality per 100 000 live births between 2016 and 2019 in rural versus urban areas.

Results. From 2016 to 2019, there was no significant increase in age-standardized rates of maternal ICU admissions in rural (170.6–192.3) or urban (161.7–172.4) areas, with a significantly higher rate, albeit a relatively small difference, in rural versus urban areas (2019 RR = 1.14; 95% confidence interval [CI] = 1.04, 1.20). Maternal mortality increased in both rural (66.9–81.7 deaths per 100 000 live births) and urban (38.1–42.3) areas and was nearly 2 times higher in rural areas (2019 RR = 1.93; 95% CI = 1.71, 2.17).

Conclusions. Pregnant individuals in rural areas are at higher risk for ICU admission and mortality than are their urban counterparts. Significant increases in maternal mortality occurred in rural and urban areas.

Public Health Implications. Public health efforts need to focus on resource-limited rural areas to mitigate geographic disparities in maternal morbidity and mortality. (*Am J Public Health*. 2023;113(2): 224–227. https://doi.org/10.2105/AJPH.2022.307134)

AJPH February 2023, Vol 113, No. 2

Although maternal mortality rates have decreased globally, those in the United States have increased significantly and now are the highest among developed countries.[1] In the United States, there are substantial place-based disparities in maternal morbidity and mortality. Data from the National Inpatient Sample from 2007 to 2015 demonstrated that rural residents had a 9% higher probability of severe maternal morbidity and mortality than did urban residents, even after controlling for socioeconomic factors and clinical conditions.[2] These data, however, do not capture individuals with out-of-hospital births, which was 1 of every 62 births in 2017 and disproportionately occurred in rural areas. Thus the differences for the overall birthing population may not be understood.[3] Additionally, those admitted to an intensive care unit (ICU) during delivery have among the most severe delivery complications, and these instances are associated with a 4 times higher increase in health care costs.[4,5] To inform strategies to mitigate this growing public health crisis, we aimed to describe contemporary rates of maternal ICU admissions and maternal mortality among pregnant individuals residing in rural compared with urban areas in the United States.

METHODS

We performed a serial cross-sectional analysis comparing rural and urban areas in the United States from 2016 to 2019 using the Centers for Disease Control and Prevention (CDC) Wide-Ranging Online Data for Epidemiologic Research (WONDER). Maternal ICU admissions were indicated on the birth certificate after delivery, and we determined maternal deaths by using *International Classification of Diseases, 10th Revision* (Geneva, Switzerland: World Health Organization; 1992) codes for pregnancy, childbirth, and the puerperium (O00-O99) as underlying or contributing cause of death.

Our analysis began with 2016, which was the first year ICU admissions were publicly available and implementation of the pregnancy-associated mortality checkbox became near universal across the United States. For each of the study years, we obtained counts of maternal ICU admissions and deaths for individuals aged 15 to 44 years in 5-year age groups stratified by rural and urban residence. We classified areas as rural or urban using the 2013 National Center for Health Statistics Classification.[6] We calculated age-standardized rates per 100 000 live births and rate ratios (RRs) using the age distribution of pregnant individuals who had a live birth in 2016, the first year of the study, by 5-year age groups.

We analyzed trends between 2016 and 2019 by estimating the average annual percentage change (AAPC) using the Joinpoint Regression Program (National Cancer Institute, Bethesda, MD). We performed all other analyses in SAS Enterprise Guide version 7.1 (SAS Institute, Cary, NC) and Stata version 14 (StataCorp LP, College Station, TX).

RESULTS

From 2016 to 2019, there were 15 295 384 live births to individuals aged 15 to 44 years. Of these births, 13.5% were to individuals residing in rural areas and 86.5% in urban areas. Self-reported race and ethnicity were as follows: 52.7% non-Hispanic White, 15.2% non-Hispanic Black, 23.4% Hispanic, and 7.0% Asian/Pacific Islander. Compared with urban areas, rural areas had a higher proportion of pregnant individuals who were younger than 25 years (66.5% vs 51.6%), were non-Hispanic White (73.3% vs 49.4%), and had a high school education or less (47.6% vs 38.2%). The timing of prenatal care initiation was similar in both rural and urban areas, with the majority of pregnant individuals receiving care within the first 5 months.

From 2016 to 2019, there were 25 541 maternal ICU admissions during the delivery hospitalization, of which 13.9% occurred among individuals residing in rural areas (n = 3562) and 86.1% in urban areas (n = 21 979). Rates increased nonsignificantly from 170.6 (158.8–182.7) to 192.3 (179.5–205.0) ICU admissions per 100 000 live births for pregnant individuals in rural areas (AAPC+3.3%/year = –5.3%, 12.7%) and from 161.7 (157.4–165.9) to 172.4 (167.9–176.9) ICU admissions per 100 000 live births in urban areas (AAPC+2.1%/year = –3.9%, 8.5%) from 2016 to 2019 (Table 1). Rural rates in each year of the study period were between 10% and 20% significantly higher than were those in urban rates (Table 1; pooled 2016–2019 RR = 1.14; 95% confidence intervals [CI] = 1.09, 1.18).

Of the 6758 pregnancy-related deaths from 2016 to 2019, 20.4% (n = 1378) were in rural areas and 79.5% (n = 5380) in urban areas. Rates of maternal mortality per 100 000 live births increased from 2016 to 2019 in rural (from 66.9; 95% CI = 59.1, 74.6 to 81.7; CI = 73.2, 90.1; AAPC = 7.0%/year; range = 2.2%–12.1%) and urban (from 38.1; 95% CI = 36.0, 40.2 to 42.3; 95% CI = 40.1, 44.5; AAPC = 3.5%/year; range = 2.2%–12.1%) areas (Table 1). Maternal mortality rates were persistently higher among individuals in rural than in urban areas (Table 1; e.g., 2019 RR = 1.93; 95% CI = 1.71, 2.17).

DISCUSSION

In this nationwide, population-based study of adverse maternal outcomes, we found significantly higher rates of maternal ICU admissions and maternal mortality in rural than in urban areas.

TABLE 1— Comparison of Maternal Mortality and Maternal Intensive Care Unit Admissions in Rural Versus Urban Areas: United States, 2016–2019

Year	Rural, ASR (95% CI) or AAPC (Range)	Urban, ASR (95% CI) or AAPC (Range)	RR (95% CI)
Maternal ICU admission			
2016	170.6 (158.8, 182.7)	161.7 (157.4, 165.9)	1.06 (0.98, 1.14)
2017	192.2 (179.3, 205.1)	158.7 (154.5, 163.0)	1.21 (1.13, 1.30)
2018	187.4 (174.7, 200.1)	160.7 (156.4, 165.0)	1.17 (1.08, 1.25)
2019	192.3 (179.5, 205.0)	172.4 (167.9, 176.9)	1.12 (1.04, 1.20)
Pooled 2016–2019	185.5 (179.3, 191.9)	163.3 (161.2, 165.5)	1.14 (1.09, 1.18)
AAPC 2016–2019	+3.3 (-5.3 to 12.7)	+2.1% (-3.9 to 8.5)	NA
Maternal mortality			
2016	66.9 (59.1, 74.6)	38.1 (36.0, 40.2)	1.75 (1.54, 1.99)
2017	69.1 (61.4, 76.8)	39.7 (37.6, 41.9)	1.74 (1.53, 1.97)
2018	73.9 (65.8, 82.0)	40.9 (38.7, 43.1)	1.81 (1.59, 2.04)
2019	81.7 (73.2, 90.1)	42.3 (40.1, 44.5)	1.93 (1.71, 2.17)
Pooled 2016–2019	72.9 (68.9, 77.0)	40.2 (39.2, 41.3)	1.81 (1.70, 1.93)
AAPC 2016–2019	+7.0 (2.2 to 12.1)	+3.5 (2.2 to 12.1)	NA

Note. AAPC = annual average percentage change; ASR = age-standardized rate (per 100 000 live births); CI = confidence interval; ICU = intensive care unit; NA = not applicable; RR = rate ratio.

Specifically, pregnant individuals residing in rural areas experienced maternal mortality rates of up to almost twice the rate of individuals in urban areas, with persistent differences between 2016 and 2019. Moreover, in both rural and urban areas, maternal mortality rates have steadily increased.

Our findings extend those of previous studies, as we used more contemporary data using all births and pregnancy-associated deaths between 2016 and 2019. Also, previous studies analyzed rural–urban disparities in maternal morbidity and mortality as a composite measure or selected a small, subnational region for their study focus.[2,7,8] We newly provide data specifically on maternal ICU admissions from all live births as an indicator that individuals needed the highest acuity of care. Of note, the frequency of ICU admission was relatively flat and the rural–urban disparity was relatively narrow. By contrast, we demonstrated significant increases in maternal mortality rates in all geographic locales and persistent differences in the rates for rural versus urban areas.[2,7]

Although the reasons for the higher rates of adverse maternal outcomes in rural areas are likely multifactorial, substantial declines in hospital-based obstetric services between 2014 and 2018 in rural counties highlight the importance of policy efforts to ensure access to high-quality and high-acuity care.[9] Previous work has also demonstrated rural–urban differences in individual cardiovascular health factors that may contribute to adverse maternal outcomes, such as obesity, diabetes, and hypertension, as well as adverse pregnancy outcomes, such as hypertensive disorders of pregnancy.[10,11]

Limitations of this study include potential miscoding of adverse maternal outcomes on birth and death certificates as well as the potential for variation in the threshold for ICU admission between hospitals. As maternal mortality review committees are not universally available in each jurisdiction to adjudicate deaths, a more advanced understanding of causes of death is not possible with the current data set. However, the CDC WONDER Natality and Mortality Databases provide comprehensive and robust data on total maternal mortality and ICU admissions in the United States.

PUBLIC HEALTH IMPLICATIONS

Our results demonstrate higher maternal ICU admission and mortality rates in rural than in urban areas, with statistically significant increases in maternal mortality in all areas between 2016 and 2019. The disproportionate burden of maternal risk in rural areas is especially concerning given the decline of health care facilities and obstetric care in these areas. These data reflect the pervasiveness of poor maternal outcomes across the United States, and future research should incorporate the intersection of place with other important social determinants of health.[12]

Lack of access or additional barriers to abortion care are associated with adverse maternal outcomes, which suggests that future trends in maternal ICU admission and mortality rates will likely accelerate following the US Supreme Court's revocation of the constitutional right to abortion. It remains to be determined how this will differentially affect rural and urban areas and should be an area of future research. The persistent outcome gap between rural and urban areas demonstrates the added burden in resource-limited rural areas that warrant targeted public health interventions. *AJPH*

ABOUT THE AUTHORS

Katharine A. Harrington is with the Department of Preventive Medicine, Northwestern University Feinberg School of Medicine, Chicago, IL. Natalie A. Cameron is with the Division of General Internal Medicine, Northwestern University Feinberg School of Medicine. Kasen Culler is with the Department of Medicine, Northwestern University Feinberg School of Medicine. William A. Grobman is with the Department of Obstetrics and Gynecology, Ohio State University School of Medicine, Columbus. Sadiya S. Khan is with the Division of Cardiology, Northwestern University Feinberg School of Medicine.

CORRESPONDENCE

Correspondence should be sent to Sadiya S. Khan, MD, MSc, 680 N. Lakeshore Dr, Suite 1400, Chicago, IL 60611 (e-mail: s-khan-1@northwestern.edu). Reprints can be ordered at http://www.ajph.org by clicking the "Reprints" link.

PUBLICATION INFORMATION

Full Citation: Harrington KA, Cameron NA, Culler K, Grobman WA, Khan SS. Rural–urban disparities in adverse maternal outcomes in the United States, 2016–2019. *Am J Public Health*. 2023; 113(2):224–227.

Acceptance Date: September 19, 2022.

DOI: https://doi.org/10.2105/AJPH.2022.307134

CONTRIBUTORS

K. A. Harrington completed the analyses and the first draft of the article. K. A. Harrington and S. S. Khan designed the study. N. A. Cameron, K. Culler, W. A. Grobman, and S. S Khan made critical revisions to the article. N. A. Cameron, W. A. Grobman, and S. S Khan supervised the analyses and contributed to the interpretation of the findings.

ACKNOWLEDGMENTS

S. S. Khan received funding from the National Heart, Lung, and Blood Institute, National Institutes of Health (NIH; grant NHLBI HL161514).

Note. The content of this research brief is solely the responsibility of the authors and does not necessarily represent the official views of the NIH.

CONFLICTS OF INTEREST

The authors have no conflicts of interest to declare.

HUMAN PARTICIPANT PROTECTION

The Northwestern University Feinberg School of Medicine institutional review board deemed this study exempt from review because of the publicly available de-identified nature of the data used.

REFERENCES

1. Hirshberg A, Srinivas SK. Epidemiology of maternal morbidity and mortality. *Semin Perinatol.* 2017;41(6):332–337. https://doi.org/10.1053/j.semperi.2017.07.007
2. Kozhimannil KB, Interrante JD, Henning-Smith C, Admon LK. Rural-urban differences in severe maternal morbidity and mortality in the US, 2007–15. *Health Aff (Millwood).* 2019;38(12):2077–2085. https://doi.org/10.1377/hlthaff.2019.00805
3. MacDorman MF, Declercq E. Trends and state variations in out-of-hospital births in the United States, 2004–2017. *Birth.* 2019;46(2):279–288. https://doi.org/10.1111/birt.12411
4. Obstetric care consensus no. 5: severe maternal morbidity: screening and review. *Obstet Gynecol.* 2016;128(3):e54–e60. https://doi.org/10.1097/AOG.0000000000001642
5. Debbink MP, Metz TD, Nelson RE, et al. Directly measured costs of severe maternal morbidity events during delivery admission compared with uncomplicated deliveries. *Am J Perinatol.* 2022;39(6):567–576. https://doi.org/10.1055/s-0041-1740237
6. Ingram DD, Franco SJ. 2013 NCHS urban–rural classification scheme for counties. *Vital Health Stat 2.* 2014;(166):1–73.
7. Merkt PT, Kramer MR, Goodman DA, et al. Urban-rural differences in pregnancy-related deaths, United States, 2011–2016. *Am J Obstet Gynecol.* 2021;225(2):183.e1–183.e16. https://doi.org/10.1016/j.ajog.2021.02.028
8. Hansen A, Moloney M. Pregnancy-related mortality and severe maternal morbidity in rural Appalachia: established risks and the need to know more. *J Rural Health.* 2020;36(1):3–8. https://doi.org/10.1111/jrh.12383
9. Kozhimannil KB, Interrante JD, Tuttle MKS, Henning-Smith C. Changes in hospital-based obstetric services in rural US counties, 2014–2018. *JAMA.* 2020;324(2):197–199. https://doi.org/10.1001/jama.2020.5662
10. Centers for Disease Control and Prevention. Obesity prevalence among adults living in metropolitan and nonmetropolitan counties—United States, 2016. *MMWR Morb Mortal Wkly Rep.* 2018;67(23):653–658. http://dx.doi.org/10.15585/mmwr.mm6723a1
11. Mainous AG 3rd, King DE, Garr DR, Pearson WS. Race, rural residence, and control of diabetes and hypertension. *Ann Fam Med.* 2004;2(6):563–568. https://doi.org/10.1370/afm.119
12. Centers for Disease Control and Prevention. Vital signs: pregnancy-related deaths, United States, 2011–2015, and strategies for prevention, 13 states, 2013–2017. *MMWR Morb Mortal Wkly Rep.* 2019;68(18):423–429. https://doi.org/10.15585/mmwr.mm6818e1

The COVID-19 Pandemic, Socioeconomic Effects, and Intimate Partner Violence Against Women: A Population-Based Cohort Study in 2020, Iran

Reza Fereidooni, MD, Jennifer Mootz, PhD, Rasoul Sabaei, MS, Kaveh Khoshnood, PhD, MPH, Seyed Taghi Heydari, PhD, Mohammad Javad Moradian, MD, PhD, MPH, Erfan Taherifard, MD, Maryam Nasirian, PhD, and Hossein Molavi Vardanjani, PhD, MPH

See also Alang and Blackstock, p. 194, Ferreira and Buttell, p. 136, and Kapadia, p. 144.

Objectives. To investigate the prevalence, pattern, and socioeconomic risk factors of intimate partner violence (IPV) before and 6 months after the pandemic onset among a cohort of Iranian women.

Methods. We conducted a population-based IPV survey among 2502 partnered Iranian women aged 18 to 60 years before (n = 2502) and 6 months after (n=2116) the pandemic's onset. We estimated prevalence and incidence of psychological, physical, and sexual IPV, and the odds of different forms of IPV associated with main exposure variables, adjusted for participant relationship factors.

Results. Pandemic prevalence of IPV (65.4%; 95% confidence interval [CI] = 63.4%, 67.4%) was higher than prepandemic prevalence (54.2%; 95% CI = 52.2%, 56.3%). At follow-up, the incidence of IPV was 25.5% (95% CI = 22.9%, 28.4%). The highest incidence was in cases of physical and sexual IPV. Women whose partners lost their employment were at significant risk of new exposure to IPV. Highest socioeconomic status (SES) was associated with less physical IPV (odds ratio = 0.03; 95% CI = 0.01, 0.14).

Conclusions. IPV prevalence has risen since the COVID-19 epidemic began with many women who had never experienced IPV now facing it. Unemployment of women or their partners and prepandemic lower socioeconomic status are risk factors of IPV. Monitoring programs should target these populations. (*Am J Public Health*. 2023;113(2):228–237. https://doi.org/10.2105/AJPH.2022.306839)

AJPH February 2023, Vol 113, No. 2

Intimate partner violence (IPV) against women is a challenging and preventable global health concern.[1] IPV can cause a wide range of negative outcomes, including acute traumatic injuries, mental illnesses, decreased quality of life, and even premature death.[2,3]

According to reports published worldwide, IPV against women has sharply increased in the era of the COVID-19 pandemic.[4,5] Porter et al. performed a telephone survey in Peru, questioning a cohort about their experiences with physical IPV throughout the lockdown period. Comparing the newly collected data with those from their last round of data collection in 2016, they found an 8.3% increase in reported physical violence within households.[6] In a cross-sectional study in Ethiopia, the prevalence of IPV during COVID-19 pandemic restrictions was 22.4%, which is close to the national prepandemic figures.[7] A cross-sectional survey conducted by Hamadani et al. in Bangladesh revealed a significant decrease in the economic and psychosocial well-being of women since the lockdown, with over half of participants reporting "more frequent" IPV than in the prelockdown era.[8] Several other reports have also demonstrated a surge in IPV.[9] Furthermore, the number of calls to hotlines has decreased in some contexts where IPV victims were unable to call because they had been confined with their abusive partner during the stay-at-home order.[5] These reports highlight the urgency of conducting systematic studies that actively survey women to investigate the effects of the COVID-19 pandemic on IPV instead of merely relying on hotline call data.

Although the most significant risk factors of IPV are well established, it is less clear who is at increased risk of experiencing IPV during a social and public health crisis, such as the COVID-19 pandemic.[10] During the first months of the epidemic, a large number of people lost their jobs and some fell into poverty for the first time.[11,12] This newfound position could be stressful and result in a higher likelihood of violent behaviors.[13] The pandemic could also act through its effects on mental health. High levels of psychological distress—which have a mutual relationship with IPV—were reported during the pandemic.[14] Economically, COVID-19 has hit low- and middle-income countries particularly hard.[15] In low- and middle-income countries, a considerable portion of jobs could be lost and many people could experience poverty early during a lockdown or social-distancing situation.[16,17] Iran, a middle-income country, has experienced an extensive spread of COVID-19. Prior to the start of COVID-19, Iran was subjected to harsh unilateral economic sanctions imposed by the United States, which resulted in a dire economic situation, high inflation, and a high unemployment rate.[18] According to official reports, about 1 million jobs were lost in the first year of the pandemic, and the labor force participation rate has dropped from more than 44% to 41.3%.[19] Before the onset of COVID-19, the rate of IPV against Iranian women was more than 50%, with the most prevalent types being psychological and physical.[20,21]

No study has yet transpired to investigate the impact of the COVID-19 pandemic on different types of IPV and to determine its risk factors in a cohort group. We conducted a population-based survey on the prevalence and patterns of IPV against women soon before the start of the COVID-19 pandemic, using a standard IPV questionnaire; we were thus uniquely positioned to build a cohort of women to follow 6 months into the pandemic. We chose this time range because we could not foresee how long the epidemic would last, and 6 months is plenty of time for the pattern of IPV to have its full effect as families' finances deplete and the mental effects of the new living condition set in. Following these women allowed us to ascertain exposure rates to psychological, physical, and sexual IPV before and during the COVID-19 pandemic. To our knowledge, this is the first study to analyze rates of new exposures to different forms of IPV during COVID-19 and to use longitudinal data to identify women at higher risk of being newly exposed to IPV during the pandemic. Our study aimed to estimate the prevalence of IPV against women who stayed with the same partner 6 months into the beginning of the pandemic (hereafter, "pandemic phase"), estimate the portion who have been newly exposed to IPV (incidence) in the era of the pandemic, and investigate the effects of job loss and socioeconomic status (SES) on the prevalence and incidence of IPV against women.

METHODS

This population-based cohort study was conducted in the city of Isfahan in 2020. COVID-19 was first confirmed in Iran in February 2020, after which restrictions and mandates on closing some businesses were implemented. The employment rate in Isfahan province dropped from 41.2% in spring 2019 to 36.3% in spring 2020.[11] More information about the COVID-19 situation in the city of Isfahan can be found in the Appendix (available as a supplement to the online version of this article at http://www.ajph.org).

Study Design and Participants

We collected baseline data in a population-based survey primarily designed to estimate the prevalence of IPV in a cross-sectional study design. We collected the baseline data from January 14 to February 15, 2020, 4 days before the first cases of COVID-19 were officially confirmed in Iran. The inclusion criteria for this phase were as follows: women were 18 to 60 years old, had lived in Isfahan for at least 1 recent year, could speak Persian, and expressed informed consent to participate in the study. Considering the COVID-19 pandemic as a natural exposure, we designed a new data collection phase to be conducted 6 months after the onset of the pandemic. Women who were interviewed in our baseline phase were eligible to participate. This phase was completed from August 15 to September 14, 2020. We excluded participants who were divorced or widowed at the baseline measurement phase or during the follow-up period, as well as those who were not partnered with the same person or not interested in participating in the follow-up.

We obtained a list of all active female-owned cellphones with a residential address located in each of the different urban districts of the Isfahan metropolis. More information about cellphone number acquisition is available in the Appendix. We defined each urban district of Isfahan as a sampling stratum, and we conducted proportional-to-size sampling. We selected participants by applying a random-digit-number dialing procedure for the study's first phase;

participants were then contacted by 2 female social workers for a telephone interview. The same interviewers followed up the participants with a phone interview 6 months later.

Although extramarital relationships are already widespread and increasing in Iranian society (especially among the younger generation), they are still socioculturally unacceptable and even punishable by law.[22] For these sociocultural reasons, we were obliged to exclude women who had intimate partner relationships outside of marriage.

We calculated the sample size for our prevalence survey (prepandemic). In the prepandemic phase, 3250 calls were made. A total of 2502 women completed the prepandemic survey (response rate = 89%). Of these 2502 women, 188 were divorced or widowed before the pandemic and 14 terminated their relationship during the pandemic and thus were not eligible for follow-up. Additionally, 184 women did not participate in the follow-up survey. The final number of women who completed the pandemic phase was 2116 (Appendix, Figure A).

Data Collection

The primary outcome was the self-reported experience of IPV during the last 6 months. We measured physical (6 items), psychological (11 items), and sexual (3 items) IPV using the validated Persian version of the World Health Organization multicountry study questionnaire on women's health and domestic violence.[23,24] The questions about physical IPV assessed severe (hitting repeatedly, kicking, dragging, choking, intentional burning, and threatening with a weapon or actual use of a weapon) and moderate (slapping, pushing, and throwing objects) forms of violence. We asked participants if they had been exposed to different forms of IPV during their lifetime, the past 12 months, and the past 6 months. In this study, we analyzed data from the past 6 months. We defined severity of experience as the number of IPV types a woman was exposed to in the pandemic phase.

We obtained demographic variables for women and their partners in the prepandemic phase. These included current age, age at the beginning of the relationship, duration of the intimate relationship, cohabitation status (together or separate), education level, employment (participant = housewife, employed; partner = full-time, part-time, unemployed, other), number of children, SES, and housing occupancy status (owner, tenant, other). At follow-up, we readministered the questions on the employment status of the participant and her partner and all IPV items, and we created new variables.

We established SES level by collecting asset data using the SES questionnaire developed for the PERSIAN Cohort (Prospective Epidemiological Research Studies in IrAN).[25] More information about the SES and employment data are provided in the online Appendix.

Experienced female social workers trained to collect data in this study via a lecture, a standard interview, and 2 role-playing scenarios performed the phone interviews. In the prepandemic phase of the study, we assessed interviewers' agreement in a pilot study (n = 25; κ coefficient = 0.89). The same interviewers conducted the follow-up interviews of the pandemic phase. To improve the representativeness of our sample, 3 additional calls to reach participants who did not answer the first call were scheduled at different times. At the beginning of each interview, participants were informed of the study's purpose and provided informed verbal consent in both study phases. The participants were given time to complete any urgent tasks they were doing at the moment, then to go to a private place to answer the questions safely and calmly. They were told they could end the conversation anytime they wanted, and were assured that their answers to the questions were fully confidential. Interviews lasted for an average of 10 to 15 minutes. Further conversations with women who asked for counseling were made. At the end of each interview, the social workers provided their phone numbers and an IPV hotline number to the participants.

Statistical Analysis

We estimated prevalence and its 95% confidence interval (CI) for each type of IPV. We estimated cumulative incidence proportion of IPV (hereafter, "incidence") and its 95% CI among women with no previous exposure to IPV. We calculated relative increase as follows: [absolute excess prevalence/(prepandemic prevalence × 100)]. We applied the χ^2 test to compare IPV incidence in different subpopulations during the pandemic. We used 2 independent sample *t* tests to compare the mean of different continuous variables between those exposed to IPV during the pandemic and those not exposed. Because SES data comprised discrete variables and many qualitative variables with different assigned scales, we used multiple correspondence analysis to categorize SES (Appendix, "SES Determination and Categorization"). We applied binary logistic regression modeling to identify the independent association of main exposure variables (job loss, partner's job loss, and prepandemic SES) with the study outcomes (incidence of different forms of IPV) when adjusted for confounding variables (i.e., age, age at the beginning of the relationship, duration of the intimate relationship, cohabitation status, education level, and number of children). None of these variables were collinear, and no variable selection technique was applied. A cutoff *P* value of less than .05 indicated significance. We performed data analysis using Stata software (Release 11; StataCorp LP, College Station, TX).

RESULTS

A total of 2300 women participated in the prepandemic phase, with a follow-up rate of 92% (n = 2116; online Figure A). Participants' average age was 37.4 years. The prevalence of all types of IPV was 54.2% (95% CI = 52.2%, 56.3%) at baseline (prepandemic) and 65.4% (95% CI = 63.4%, 67.4%) 6 months into the pandemic. Employment status did not improve for any of the participants or their spouses during the pandemic. All women who had lost their job in the pandemic reported exposure to violence (Table 1).

To demonstrate which factors made women susceptible to experiencing IPV in the pandemic, we compared the mean of continuous variables between women who experienced IPV for the first time in the first 6 months of the pandemic and those who did not (Table 2). Women who experienced IPV in the pandemic were married longer and had more children.

Of women reporting no experience of IPV before the pandemic, 25.5% (95% CI = 22.9%, 28.4%) revealed that they were exposed to at least 1 episode of IPV during the first 6 months of the pandemic. Incidents accounted for 17.9% of all pandemic cases of IPV. Table 3 presents the prevalence and incidence of different types of IPV by the time of measurement.

We used multivariable logistic regression modeling to evaluate the impact of COVID-19–related fallout in different groups. We considered an exposure to each type of IPV in women not previously exposed to that type of IPV (i.e., at-risk population) to be an outcome. This model showed that the loss of employment for a woman or her spouse increased her chances of being exposed to IPV (for women, adjusted odds ratio [AOR] = 355.35; 95% CI = 127.2, 993; for spouses, AOR = 342.44; 95% CI = 33.19, 3533.51). This increase is especially discernible in the case of psychological IPV (AOR = 23.72; 95% CI = 13.36, 42.12). On the other hand, physical IPV is a major issue in women with low SES (OR = 32.94; 95% CI = 7.07, 153.49). Table 4 presents associated factors of experiencing different types of IPV among women who were not exposed before the pandemic.

DISCUSSION

To our knowledge, this is one of the first longitudinal studies globally to investigate the prevalence and severity of IPV against women before and during the COVID-19 pandemic. Our study of 2116 women in Isfahan, Iran showed that the prevalence of IPV increased to more than 65% (relative increase = 21%). We also demonstrated that 25.5% of women with no previous experience of IPV before the pandemic were newly exposed to IPV during the first 6 months of the pandemic. Having a low to moderate SES at baseline, loss of the woman's job, and negative changes in the employment status of the woman's partner (job loss or demotion) were associated with being newly exposed to IPV.

Hamadani et al.[8] reported a similar increase in IPV incidence during the first month of the pandemic in a rural area in Bangladesh; they had to rely on participants retrospectively reporting their IPV experiences. Most available evidence is not population-based but generated from surveillance data from IPV hotlines. Major metropolitan areas in the United States, for instance, have observed an increase in IPV hotline calls since the onset of the COVID-19 outbreak, whereas a decrease in the number of calls has occurred in other US cities.[5,26] Such decreases are likely because of a rise in underreporting IPV due to having to quarantine with violent partners and not having private locations to call for help. Our study differs from studies based on the hotline data in that we actively reached women and, by doing a telephone survey, we reached those who may not have been informed about the existence of a hotline or those who would not want to call a hotline as they believed it would not be of use.

We also found significant associations between SES and employment loss and the risk of exposure to IPV. Women with a low or middle SES were at higher risk of more exposure to IPV during the pandemic. Many middle- and low-SES families were rental tenants who might have experienced greater housing insecurity in addition to other stressors. In Iran, the cost of living and rent during the pandemic has increased markedly.[27] Consequently, it can be deduced that a portion of families have been forced to live in smaller houses and relocate to lower-income urban neighborhoods. Middle- and low-SES families may have had less savings to buffer the effects of the slowing economy.[28] Furthermore, women who had partners who lost

TABLE 1— Characteristics of Women Who Experienced Any Type of Intimate Partner Violence (IPV) Before and During the COVID-19 Pandemic: Isfahan, Iran, 2020

Characteristics	Prepandemic (n = 2300), No. (%)	Those Lost to Follow-Up (n = 184), No. (%)	All Participants With Completed Follow-Up (n = 2116)		At-Risk Participants With Completed Follow-Up (n = 972)[a]		P
			No. (%)	IPV Prevalence (95% CI)	No. (%)	IPV Incidence (95% CI)	
Woman's age, y							.67
18–29	564 (24.5)	33 (17.9)	531 (25.1)	57.8 (53.6, 62.0)	283 (29.1)	20.8 (16.3, 26.1)	
30–39	913 (39.7)	127 (69.0)	786 (37.1)	69.1 (65.8, 72.2)	339 (34.9)	29.8 (25.0, 35.0)	
40–49	466 (20.2)	10 (5.4)	456 (21.5)	62. 9 (58.4, 67.3)	218 (22.4)	23.4 (17.9, 29.6)	
50–60	357 (15.5)	14 (7.6)	343 (16.2)	72 (67.0, 76.5)	132 (13.6)	28.0 (20.6, 36.5)	
Woman's education							.011
Illiterate	263 (11.4)	13 (7.0)	250 (11.8)	73.2 (67.4, 78.3)	101 (10.4)	34.7 (25.5, 44.8)	
Up to diploma	862 (37.5)	77 (41.8)	785 (37.1)	68.4 (65.1, 71.6)	356 (36.6)	31.2 (26.4, 36.3)	
Post-diploma to bachelor	819 (35.6)	75 (40.7)	744 (32.3)	63.6 (60.1, 67.0)	337 (34.7)	20.5 (16.3, 25.2)	
Master's degree or more	356 (15.5)	19 (10.3)	337 (15.9)	56.7 (51.3, 61.9)	178 (18.3)	18.5 (13.1, 25.0)	
Woman's job							< .001
Housework	1512 (65.7)	98 (53.2)	1414 (66.8)	67.9 (65.4, 70.3)	656 (67.5)	31.6 (28.0, 35.3)	
Employed	788 (34.2)	86 (46.7)	702 (33.2)	60.4 (56.7, 64.0)	316 (32.5)	13.0 (9.5, 17.2)	
Change in woman's job status							< .001
Remained employed	NA	NA	702 (33.2)	60.4 (56.7, 64.0)	316 (32.5)	13.0 (9.5, 17.2)	
Became unemployed	NA	NA	31 (1.5)	100 (88.8, 100)	31 (3.2)	100 (88.8, 100)	
Remained a housewife	NA	NA	1383 (65.3)	67.2 (64.7, 69.6)	625 (64.3)	28.2 (24.7, 31.9)	
SES							< .001
Low	548 (23.8)	41 (22.2)	507 (24.0)	76.5 (72.6, 80)	196 (20.2)	41.3 (34.4, 48.6)	
Low-middle	652 (28.3)	52 (28.2)	600 (28.3)	66.2 (62.3, 69.8)	274 (28.2)	25.9 (20.8, 31.5)	
Middle-high	590 (25.6)	50 (27.1)	540 (25.5)	63.1 (59, 67.1)	262 (26.9)	24.0 (19.0, 29.7)	
High	510 (22.2)	41 (22.2)	469 (22.2)	55 (50.5, 59.5)	240 (24.7)	13.8 (9.7, 18.77)	
Spouse's age, y							.12
18–29	222 (9.6)	21 (11.4)	201 (9.5)	46.3 (39.5, 53.2)	133 (13.7)	18.8 (12.5, 26.5)	
30–39	899 (39.0)	105 (57.0)	794 (37.5)	67 (63.7, 70.2)	342 (35.2)	24.6 (20.1, 29.5)	
40–49	626 (27.2)	34 (18.4)	592 (28.0)	66.4 (62.5, 70.1)	277 (28.5)	28.9 (23.6, 34.6)	
50–59	300 (13.0)	10 (5.4)	290 (13.7)	64.1 (58.4, 69.4)	142 (14.6)	28.2 (20.9, 36.3)	
≥ 60	253 (11.0)	14 (7.6)	239 (11.3)	75.3 (69.4, 80.4)	78 (8.0)	24.4 (15.3, 35.4)	
Spouse's job							< .001
Full-time	1417 (61.6)	119 (64.6)	1182 (55.8)	56.1 (53.2, 58.9)	554 (57.0)	6.9 (4.9, 9.3)	

Continued

TABLE 1— Continued

Characteristics	Prepandemic (n = 2300), No. (%)	Those Lost to Follow-Up (n = 184), No. (%)	All Participants With Completed Follow-Up (n = 2116)		At-Risk Participants With Completed Follow-Up (n = 972)[a]		P
			No. (%)	IPV Prevalence (95% CI)	No. (%)	IPV Incidence (95% CI)	
Part-time	643 (27.9)	46 (25.0)	577 (27.3)	77.1 (73.5, 80.4)	190 (19.6)	32.1 (25.5, 39.2)	
Unemployed	86 (3.7)	6 (3.2)	210 (9.9)	84.8 (79.2, 89.0)	152 (15.6)	79.6 (72.3, 85.7)	
Other	154 (6.7)	13 (7.0)	147 (6.9)	66.7 (58.6, 73.8)	76 (7.8)	36.8 (26.1, 48.7)	
Change in spouse's job status							< .001
Full-time remained full-time	NA	NA	1182 (55.9)	56.1(53.2, 58.9)	554 (57.0)	6.9 (4.9, 9.3)	
Full-time became part-time or unemployed	NA	NA	116 (5.5)	96.6 (91.2, 98.7)	116 (11.9)	96.6 (91.4, 99.1)	
Part-time remained part-time	NA	NA	559 (26.4)	76.4 (72.7, 79.7)	172 (17.7)	25.0 (18.7, 32.2)	
Part-time became unemployed	NA	NA	47 (2.2)	78.7 (64.8, 88.2)	47 (4.8)	78.7 (64.3, 89.3)	
Unemployed remained unemployed	NA	NA	80 (3.8)	77.5 (67.1, 85.3)	22 (2.3)	22.7 (7.8, 45.4)	
Other	NA	NA	132 (6.2)	62.9 (54.3, 70.7)	61 (6.3)	21.3 (11.9, 33.7)	
Spouse's education							.009
Illiterate	300 (13.0)	18 (9.7)	282 (13.3)	71.3 (65.7, 76.3)	117 (12.0)	30.8 (22.6, 40.0)	
Up to diploma	756 (32.8)	64 (34.7)	692 (32.7)	68.6 (65.1, 72.0)	315 (32.4)	31.7 (26.6, 37.2)	
Post-diploma or more	1244 (54.0)	102 (55.4)	1142 (54.0)	62 (59.1, 64.8)	540 (55.6)	20.7 (17.4, 24.4)	

Note. CI = confidence interval; NA = not applicable; SES = socioeconomic status.
[a]At risk for any new IPV experience during the first 6 months of the pandemic.

employment were at higher risk of being newly exposed to IPV.

None of the women whose husbands or themselves lost their jobs reported prepandemic IPV. Even though it is unlikely that these groups had indeed never been exposed to violence, one can rationalize that these groups stayed away from significant violence until unemployment—a major risk factor—was introduced. Also, because we do not see this zero prepandemic violence in the larger subgroups, we can assume that sparse data bias may have contributed to this finding. Moreover, all women who were employed before the pandemic but lost their employment during the pandemic reported that they experienced IPV; this may be because these women were not accustomed to staying at home, and the extra time they spent with their partner resulted in conflict. Tension resulting from spending extra time with a newly unemployed partner may be one of the reasons violence increased among women whose partners or themselves lost employment. A fascinating finding is that the spouses' job loss was more influential than women's job status change, which can be explained by men in Iranian households being the primary breadwinners.

The pattern of IPV varies in different SES groups. As shown in Table 4, although chances of experiencing psychological violence vary only slightly in the different SES subgroups, lower SES was associated with a significantly higher chance of sexual and physical violence. This may stem from the lower-class culture, where some traditional or oppressive beliefs regarding women still exist that entitle men to perpetuate and compel women to accept physical and sexual violence. It is also possible that women from higher

AJPH February 2023, Vol 113, No. 2

TABLE 2— Mean of Continuous Variables Among Women Who Were Exposed to Intimate Partner Violence (IPV) for the First Time During the Pandemic Versus Those Who Were Not: Isfahan, Iran, 2020

	Any IPV, Mean (95% CI)			Physical IPV, Mean (95% CI)			Psychological IPV, Mean (95% CI)			Sexual IPV, Mean (95% CI)		
Factor	Not Exposed After Start of Pandemic (n = 724)	Exposed During First 6 Months of Pandemic (n = 248)	P	Not Exposed After Start of Pandemic (n = 1,649)	Exposed During First 6 Months of Pandemic (n = 125)	P	Not Exposed After Start of Pandemic (n = 920)	Exposed During First 6 Months of Pandemic (n = 159)	P	Not Exposed After Start of Pandemic (n = 1600)	Exposed During First 6 Months of Pandemic (n = 146)	P
Current age, y	36.31 (35.56, 37.05)	37.61 (36.38, 38.85)	.08	37.01 (36.52, 37.50)	37.59 (35.98, 39.20)	.53	36.68 (36.02, 37.34)	37.45 (35.94, 38.97)	.38	37.78 (37.27, 38.29)	36.57 (34.96, 38.18)	.18
Age at marriage, y	24.08 (23.64, 24.53)	23.56 (22.90, 24.21)	.22	23.65 (23.37, 23.93)	23.13 (22.32, 23.93)	.33	23.86 (23.47, 24.24)	24.03 (23.19, 24.87)	.73	23.80 (23.52, 24.09)	23.71 (22.87, 24.54)	.84
Marriage duration, y	12.22 (14.37, 15.64)	14.06 (12.72, 15.39)	.022	13.36 (12.83, 13.90)	14.46 (12.93, 16.22)	.28	12.82 (12.1, 13.54)	13.42 (11.78, 15.06)	.53	13.98 (13.42, 14.54)	12.86 (11.24, 14.48)	.26
No. of children	2.24 (2.17, 2.32)	2.48 (2.35, 2.60)	.003	2.36 (2.31, 2.41)	2.64 (2.33, 2.43)	.004	2.34 (2.27, 2.40)	2.38 (2.21, 2.54)	.63	2.40 (2.35, 2.45)	2.40 (2.23, 2.57)	> .99
Age difference with spouse, y	1.89 (1.86, 1.93)	1.89 (1.83, 1.94)	.83	1.93 (1.90, 1.95)	1.95 (1.85, 2.05)	.58	1.91 (1.87, 1.94)	1.89 (1.87, 1.94)	.64	1.92 (1.89, 1.94)	1.88 (1.79, 1.96)	.37

Note. CI = confidence interval.

SES were more reluctant to admit to receiving physical or sexual violence because it is more taboo and harder to accept in their general milieu.

Women newly exposed to IPV may be unaware of how to access and utilize available services, a situation that puts them at a higher risk for repeated IPV exposures.[29] The recent exposure to economic stressors and employment loss could strain communication and interactions in intimate relationships when both partners are at home together without social or vocational social support.[4,30] Accordingly, more focused IPV screening should target families in which one or both partners have lost their jobs.

Nationwide or multination studies can further prove the impact of the COVID-19 pandemic on domestic violence in lower-income settings. However, Isfahan can act as a standard metropolis with similar features to most other metropolises in Iran, as it has a similar male-to-female ratio, age, religion, and income composition.[31] Furthermore, given that in our sampling method women from different social backgrounds were included, we believe these reports are generalizable to women residing in Iranian urban areas, especially metropolises, and by extension to other countries with similar income brackets and similar sociocultural values—for example, low-income and middle-low-income countries with traditional Middle Eastern or Islamic culture.

Recently, strategies have been proposed to address the so-called hidden crisis of IPV embedded within the COVID-19 pandemic.[5,32–34] Many recommendations come from high-income settings. These strategies may not translate well to low-resource countries with less infrastructure to provide

TABLE 3— Prevalence, Incidence, and Pattern of Intimate Partner Violence (IPV) During the COVID-19 Pandemic: Isfahan, Iran, 2020

	Prevalence During First 6 Months of Pandemic (n = 2116), % (95% CI)	Relative Increase (% of Prepandemic Prevalence)	At-Risk Participants (n = 2116), No. (%) of Completed Follow-Ups	Incidence During First 6 Months of Pandemic, % (95% CI)
Type of IPV				
Any	65.4 (63.3, 67.4)	21	972 (45.9)	25.5 (22.9, 28.4)
Physical	21.1 (19.5, 22.9)	33	1774 (83.8)	7.0 (5.9, 8.3)
Moderate physical	17.7 (16.1, 19.4)	34	1995 (94.3)	5.4 (4.5, 6.5)
Severe physical	3.6 (2.9, 4.5)	33	2060 (97.4)	1.2 (0.8, 1.8)
Psychological	56.2 (54.1, 58.3)	12.2	1079 (51.0)	14.7 (12.7, 17.0)
Sexual	23.5 (21.7, 25.3)	34	1746 (82.5)	8.3 (7.1, 9.7)
Severity of experience[a]				
1 type	37.6 (35.5, 39.7)	16.1	972 (45.9)	22.3 (19.8, 25.1)
2 types	20.2 (18.5, 21.9)	33.4	972 (45.9)	2.8 (2.0, 4.1)
3 types	7.6 (6.5, 8.8)	13.6	972 (45.9)	0.2 (0.05, 0.8)

Note. CI = confidence interval.
[a]Severity of experience is defined as number of IPV types women were exposed to in the pandemic phase.

TABLE 4— Factors Associated With Incidence of Each Type of Intimate Partner Violence (IPV) During the Pandemic: Isfahan, Iran, 2020

Factor	IPV (n = 972),[a] AOR (95% CI)	Physical IPV (n = 1774),[a] AOR (95% CI)	Psychological IPV (n = 1079),[a] AOR (95% CI)	Sexual IPV (n = 1746),[a] AOR (95% CI)
SES				
Low	5.28 (1.93, 14.42)	32.94 (7.07, 153.49)	1.83 (0.76, 4.39)	5.03 (2.09, 12.09)
Low-middle	1.87 (0.78, 4.51)	13.76 (3.09, 61.28)	0.58 (0.27, 1.22)	4.19 (1.91, 9.19)
Middle-high	2.32 (0.98, 5.47)	9.37 (2.10, 41.87)	1.12 (0.56, 2.28)	1.87 (0.84, 4.14)
High (Ref)	1	1	1	1
Change in woman's job status				
Remained employed (Ref)	1	1	1	1
Became unemployed	342.44 (33.19, 3533.51)	1.03 (0.25, 4.17)	3.22 (1.21, 8.58)	3.50 (1.34, 9.4)
Remained housewife	3.03 (1.44, 6.43)	1.48 (0.83, 2.63)	1.15 (0.64, 2.07)	1.41 (0.84, 2.92)
Change in spouse's job status				
Full-time remained full-time (Ref)	1	1	1	1
Full-time became part-time or unemployed	355.35 (127.2, 993)	5.82 (3.12, 10.84)	23.72 (13.36, 42.12)	8.10 (4.63, 14.15)
Part-time remained part-time	2.25 (1.2, 5.8)	1.37 (0.80, 2.34)	3.06 (1.54, 6.05)	1.76 (1.05, 2.96)
Part-time became unemployed	28.62 (11.27, 72.67)	2.22 (0.89, 5.53)	19.48 (8.45, 44.92)	4.36 (1.85, 10.27)
Unemployed remained unemployed	1.42 (0.42, 4.84)	1.62 (0.62, 4.24)	1.00 (0.2, 5.06)	3.70 (1.56, 8.46)
Other	2.55 (1.11, 5.84)	1.08 (0.83, 2.63)	2.24 (0.87, 5.06)	2.08 (0.97, 4.48)

Note. AOR = adjusted odds ratio; CI = confidence interval; SES = socioeconomic status. Adjusted for participant and her partner's age, age difference between participant and her partner, participant's age at current marriage or beginning of relationship, duration of marriage or relationship, their cohabitation status, participant's educational level, and her partner's educational level.
[a]The sample sizes represent the at-risk population for incidence (new exposure) of IPV (i.e., those who had not experienced IPV at the start of the pandemic).

shelter and resources for women who choose to separate from abusive partners. Integrating national IPV guidelines into COVID-19 public health response strategies is imperative. Considering how to leverage available health care services to include IPV screening and service linkage will be instrumental. Although daily life today has changed since the pandemic's early days, the pandemic is still around, with multiple new mutations and disease peaks bringing different countries under newly imposed restrictions. Results from this study can help target the limited resources in such settings to the most vulnerable groups for screening and intervention programs to tackle domestic violence in similar health or economic crises.

Limitations

There are some limitations to this study. As in any other study using surveys, the results could be due to changes in reporting or response bias. Random digit dialing could have missed women without an active phone number. Employed or otherwise occupied women may be less likely to answer calls from unknown numbers and participate in survey interviews. IPV victims with controlling partners may have less access to their phones or private spaces. However, there was no other choice for sampling and data collection in the era of social isolation.

This study focused on the incidence of different types of IPV in women who were not exposed to IPV at baseline; however, women with persistent or worsening IPV are also relevant. The study was designed in this manner because our pilot study proved that asking women about the frequency of their experiences would result in inaccurate answers. This may be because an extended call duration puts women at risk or makes them uninterested in answering.

Conclusion

This study showed increased prevalence, incidence, and severity of IPV against women across different subpopulations in an urban setting in Iran from before COVID-19 and 6 months into the pandemic. Women at risk for being newly exposed to IPV were those who became unemployed or had partners who became unemployed or those from prepandemic middle- or low-SES households. Screening programs should target such populations in low-resource settings. Guidelines for IPV should be adapted for low- and middle-income countries and integrated into COVID-19 response plans. AJPH

ABOUT THE AUTHORS

Reza Fereidooni is with the Student Research Committee, Shiraz University of Medical Sciences, Shiraz, Iran. Jennifer Mootz is with the Department of Psychiatry, Columbia University, New York, NY. Rasoul Sabaei is with the Department of Psychology, Faculty of Psychology, Khorasgan Branch, Islamic Azad University, Isfahan, Iran. Kaveh Khoshnood is with the Yale School of Public Health, Yale University, New Haven, CT. Seyed Taghi Heydari is with the Health Policy Research Center, Institute of Health, Shiraz University of Medical Sciences, Shiraz, Iran. Mohammad Javad Moradian is with the Trauma Research Center, Shahid Rajaee (Emtiaz) Trauma Hospital, Shiraz University of Medical Sciences, Shiraz, Iran. Erfan Taherifard and Hossein Molavi Vardanjani are with the MD-MPH Program, School of Medicine, Shiraz University of Medical Sciences, Shiraz, Iran. Maryam Nasirian is with the Department of Epidemiology and Biostatistics, Health School, and Infectious Disease and Tropical Medicine Research Center, Isfahan University of Medical Sciences, Isfahan, Iran.

CORRESPONDENCE

Correspondence should be sent to Hossein Molavi Vardanjani, PhD, MPH, MPH Department, 8th Floor, 2nd Building, School of Medicine, Imam Hussain Square, Zand Street, Shiraz, 7134845794, Iran (e-mail: Molavih@sums.ac.ir, Hosseinmolavi@ymail.com). Reprints can be ordered at http://www.ajph.org by clicking the "Reprints" link.

PUBLICATION INFORMATION

Full Citation: Fereidooni R, Mootz J, Sabaei R, et al. The COVID-19 pandemic, socioeconomic effects, and intimate partner violence against women: a population-based cohort study in 2020, Iran. *Am J Public Health*. 2023;113(2):228–237.

Acceptance Date: March 8, 2022.

DOI: https://doi.org/10.2105/AJPH.2022.306839

CONTRIBUTORS

R. Fereidooni took part in data curation, the formal analysis, the investigation, the project administration, writing the original draft, and reviewing and editing the article. J. Mootz took part in conceptualization, data curation, the formal analysis, the investigation, validation, visualization, writing the original draft, and reviewing and editing the article. R. Sabaei took part in the formal analysis, project administration, resources, validation, visualization, writing the original draft, and reviewing and editing the article. K. Khoshnood took part in conceptualization, data curation, formal analysis, investigation, methodology, supervision, validation, visualization, writing the original draft, and reviewing and editing the article. S. T. Heydari took part in conceptualization, data curation, formal analysis, funding acquisition, investigation, methodology, and reviewing and editing the article. M. J. Moradian took part in project administration, resources, and reviewing and editing the article. E. Taherifard took part in the investigation, project administration, visualization, writing the original draft, and reviewing and editing the article. M. Nasirian took part in project administration, resources, and reviewing and editing the article. H. M. Vardanjani took part in conceptualization, data curation, formal analysis, funding acquisition, the investigation, methodology, project administration, resources, supervision, validation, visualization, writing the original draft, and reviewing and editing the article. R. Fereidooni, J. Mootz, K. Khoshnood, S. T. Heydari, and H. M. Vardanjani accessed and verified the data.

ACKNOWLEDGMENTS

This study is a part of the thesis project for the MD degree by R. Fereidooni. We thank Shiraz University of Medical Sciences' vice-chancellor for research that supported this work (grant number 99-01-01-23477).

A very primary draft of this work was published as a preprint at SSRN, although it has since undergone considerable revision.

We extend our sincere gratitude to the women who, sometimes despite great difficulties, participated in our study. We also thank the interviewers of our study who, with patience and precision, tried to collect quality data.

CONFLICTS OF INTEREST

The authors declare that there are no conflicts of interest.

HUMAN PARTICIPANT PROTECTION

This study was performed in accordance with the Declaration of Helsinki and was approved by the institutional review board (IRB) of Shiraz University of Medical Sciences (approval code IR.SUMS.MED.REC.1399.486). All participants provided verbal consent. Ethics board approvals were separately provided for 2 phases of studies. According to Iranian law, sharing of data containing potentially identifying or sensitive patients' information is restricted. Data are available for academic researchers via the research deputy of Shiraz Medical School (med_thesis@sums.ac.ir) upon reasonable request.

REFERENCES

1. Bair-Merritt MH. Intimate partner violence. *Pediatrics.* 2010;31(4):145–150. https://doi.org/10.1542/pir.31-4-145
2. Stockman JK, Hayashi H, Campbell JC. Intimate partner violence and its health impact on ethnic minority women. *J Womens Health (Larchmt).* 2015;24(1):62–79. https://doi.org/10.1089/jwh.2014.4879
3. Patra P, Prakash J, Patra B, Khanna P. Intimate partner violence: wounds are deeper. *Indian J Psychiatry.* 2018;60(4):494–498. https://doi.org/10.4103/psychiatry.IndianJPsychiatry_74_17
4. Bradbury-Jones C, Isham L. The pandemic paradox: the consequences of COVID-19 on domestic violence. *J Clin Nurs.* 2020;29(13–14):2047–2049. https://doi.org/10.1111/jocn.15296
5. Evans ML, Lindauer M, Farrell ME. A pandemic within a pandemic—intimate partner violence during Covid-19. *N Engl J Med.* 2020;383(24):2302–2304. https://doi.org/10.1056/NEJMp2024046
6. Porter C, Favara M, Sánchez A, Scott D. The impact of COVID-19 lockdowns on physical domestic violence: evidence from a list randomization experiment. *SSM Popul Health.* 2021;14:100792. https://doi.org/10.1016/j.ssmph.2021.100792
7. Tadesse AW, Tarekegn SM, Wagaw GB, Muluneh MD. Prevalence and associated factors of intimate partner violence among married women during COVID-19 pandemic restrictions: a community-based study. *J Interpers Violence.* 2020; Epub ahead of print. https://doi.org/10.1177/08862 60520976222
8. Hamadani JD, Hasan MI, Baldi AJ, et al. Immediate impact of stay-at-home orders to control COVID-19 transmission on socioeconomic conditions, food insecurity, mental health, and intimate partner violence in Bangladeshi women and their families: an interrupted time series. *Lancet Glob Health.* 2020; 8(11):e1380–e1389. https://doi.org/10.1016/S2214-109X(20)30366-1
9. Agüero JM. COVID-19 and the rise of intimate partner violence. *World Dev.* 2021;137:105217. https://doi.org/10.1016/j.worlddev.2020.105217
10. Capaldi DM, Knoble NB, Shortt JW, Kim HK. A systematic review of risk factors for intimate partner violence. *Partner Abuse.* 2012;3(2):231–280. https://doi.org/10.1891/1946-6560.3.2.231
11. Taherinia M, Hassanvand A. Economic consequences of Covid-19 disease on the Iranian economy; with an emphasis on employment. *Q J Nurs Manag.* 2020;9(3):43–58.
12. Martin A, Markhvida M, Hallegatte S, Walsh B. Socio-economic impacts of COVID-19 on household consumption and poverty. *Econ Disaster Clim Chang.* 2020;4(3):453–479. https://doi.org/10.1007/s41885-020-00070-3
13. Sharma A, Borah SB. Covid-19 and domestic violence: an indirect path to social and economic crisis. *J Fam Violence.* 2020:1–7. https://doi.org/10.1007/s10896-020-00188-8
14. Xiong J, Lipsitz O, Nasri F, et al. Impact of COVID-19 pandemic on mental health in the general population: a systematic review. *J Affect Disord.* 2020;277:55–64. https://doi.org/10.1016/j.jad.2020.08.001
15. Bong CL, Brasher C, Chikumba E, McDougall R, Mellin-Olsen J, Enright A. The COVID-19 pandemic: effects on low- and middle-income countries. *Anesth Analg.* 2020;131(1):86–92. https://doi.org/10.1213/ANE.0000000000004846
16. Akkermans J, Richardson J, Kraimer ML. The Covid-19 crisis as a career shock: implications for careers and vocational behavior. *J Vocat Behav.* 2020;119:103434. https://doi.org/10.1016/j.jvb.2020.103434
17. Moreira DN, Pinto da Costa M. The impact of the Covid-19 pandemic in the precipitation of intimate partner violence. *Int J Law Psychiatry.* 2020; 71:101606. https://doi.org/10.1016/j.ijlp.2020.101606
18. Abdollahi M. *Assessing the Macroeconomic Aspects of Coronavirus Outbreak.* Tehran, Iran: Islamic Parliament Research Center (IPRC) of the Islamic Republic of Iran; April 27, 2020.
19. *Detailed Results of Employment in Formal and Informal Sector 2019–2020.* Tehran, Iran: Statistical Center of Iran; October 30, 2021.
20. Hajnasiri H, Ghanei Gheshlagh R, Sayehmiri K, Moafi F, Farajzadeh M. Domestic violence among Iranian women: a systematic review and meta-analysis. *Iran Red Crescent Med J.* 2016;18(6):e34971. https://doi.org/10.5812/ircmj.34971
21. Naghavi A, Amani S, Bagheri M, De Mol J. A critical analysis of intimate partner sexual violence in Iran. *Front Psychol.* 2019;10:2729. https://doi.org/10.3389/fpsyg.2019.02729
22. Latifnejad Roudsari R, Javadnoori M, Hasanpour M, Hazavehei SMM, Taghipour A. Socio-cultural challenges to sexual health education for female adolescents in Iran. *Iran J Reprod Med.* 2013;11(2):101–110.
23. Garcia-Moreno C, Jansen HA, Ellsberg M, Heise L, Watts CH. Prevalence of intimate partner violence: findings from the WHO multi-country study on women's health and domestic violence. *Lancet.* 2006;368(9543):1260–1269. https://doi.org/10.1016/S0140-6736(06)69523-8
24. Moazen B, Salehi A, Soroush M, Molavi Vardanjani H, Zarrinhaghighi A. Domestic violence against women in Shiraz, south-western Iran. *J Inj Violence Res.* 2019;11(2):243–254. https://doi.org/10.5249/jivr.v11i2.1238
25. Poustchi H, Eghtesad S, Kamangar F, et al. Prospective epidemiological research studies in Iran (the PERSIAN Cohort Study): rationale, objectives, and design. *Am J Epidemiol.* 2018;187(4):647–655. https://doi.org/10.1093/aje/kwx314
26. Tolan C. Some cities see jumps in domestic violence during the pandemic. *CNN.* April 4, 2020. Available at: https://www.cnn.com/2020/04/04/us/domestic-violence-coronavirus-calls-cases-increase-invs/index.html. Accessed September 4, 2021.
27. *April 2020 Report on Housing Market Developments in Tehran.* Tehran, Iran: Economic Research and Policy Department, Central Bank of Iran; 2020.
28. Khoshnood A. Poverty in Iran: a critical analysis. *Middle East Policy.* 2019;26(1):60–74. https://doi.org/10.1111/mepo.12400
29. Sabri B, Huerta J, Alexander KA, St Vil NM, Campbell JC, Callwood GB. Multiple intimate partner violence experiences: knowledge, access, utilization and barriers to utilization of resources by women of the African diaspora. *J Health Care Poor Underserved.* 2015;26(4):1286–1303. https://doi.org/10.1353/hpu.2015.0135
30. Kaukinen C. When stay-at-home orders leave victims unsafe at home: exploring the risk and consequences of intimate partner violence during the COVID-19 pandemic. *Am J Crim Justice.* 2020: 45(4):668–679. https://doi.org/10.1007/s12103-020-09533-5
31. *Iran Population and Housing Census 2016 Results.* Tehran, Iran: Statistical Center of Iran; 2016.
32. Kofman YB, Garfin DR. Home is not always a haven: the domestic violence crisis amid the COVID-19 pandemic. *Psychol Trauma.* 2020;12(S1):S199–S201. https://doi.org/10.1037/tra0000866
33. van Gelder N, Peterman A, Potts A, et al. COVID-19: reducing the risk of infection might increase the risk of intimate partner violence. *EClinicalMedicine.* 2020; 21:100348. https://doi.org/10.1016/j.eclinm.2020.100348
34. Usher K, Bhullar N, Durkin J, Gyamfi N, Jackson D. Family violence and COVID-19: increased vulnerability and reduced options for support. *Int J Ment Health Nurs.* 2020;29(4):549–552. https://doi.org/10.1111/inm.12735

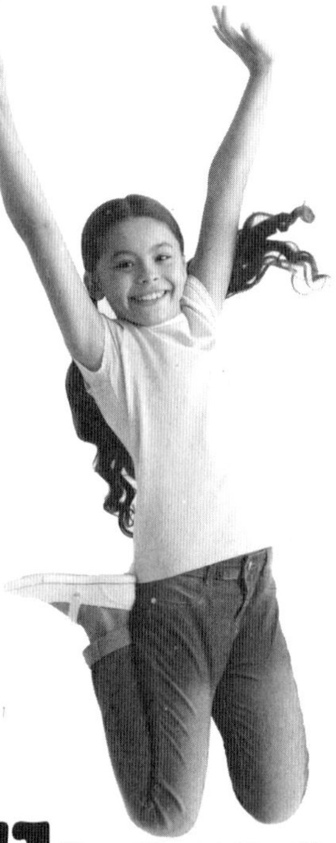

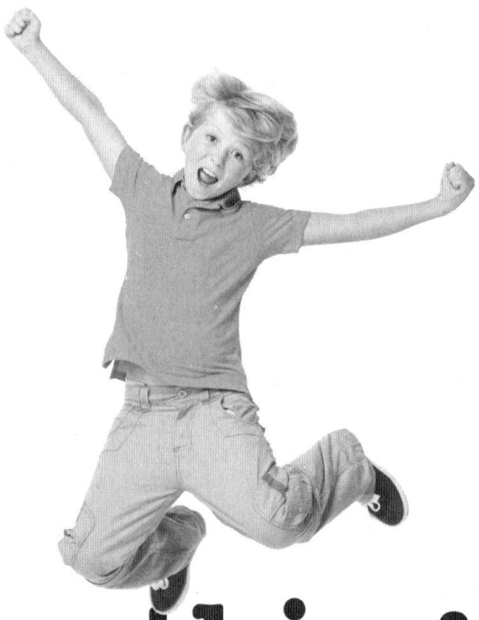

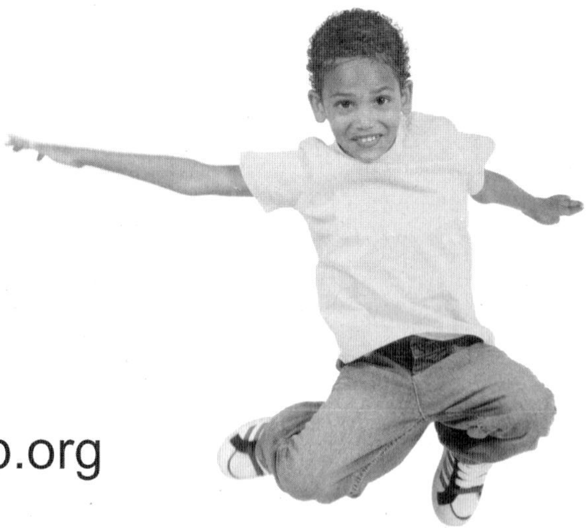

NOW IT COMES WITH A LIST OF INGREDIENTS.

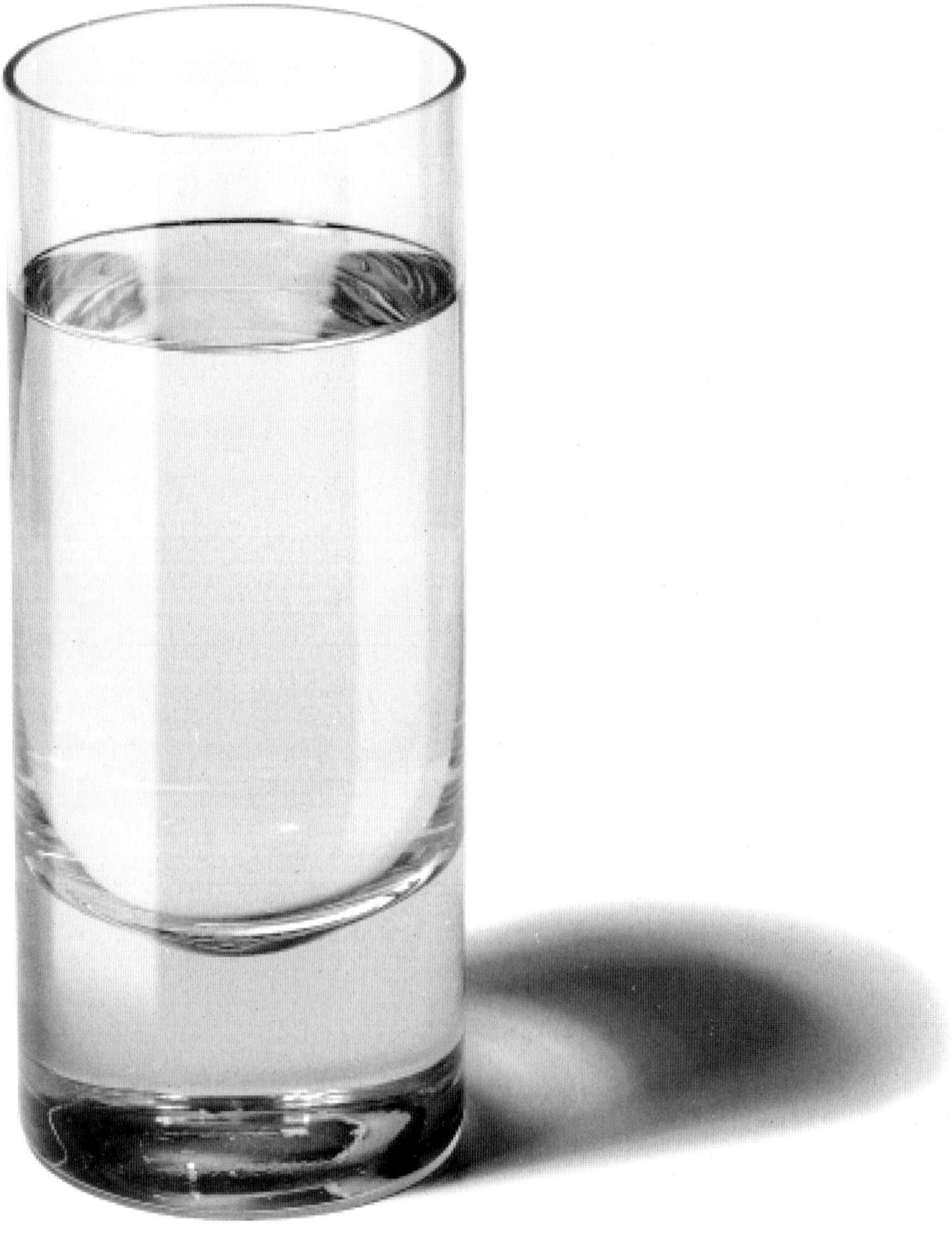

What's in your tap water besides water? A short new report from your water supplier will tell you where your water comes from, what's in it, and how safe it is. Look for the report in your mail, and read it. Because when it comes to understanding your drinking water, the most important ingredient is you.

EPA

DRINKING WATER. KNOW WHAT'S IN IT FOR YOU.

Call your water supplier or the Safe Drinking Water Hotline at 1-800-426-4791.
Or visit www.epa.gov/safewater/

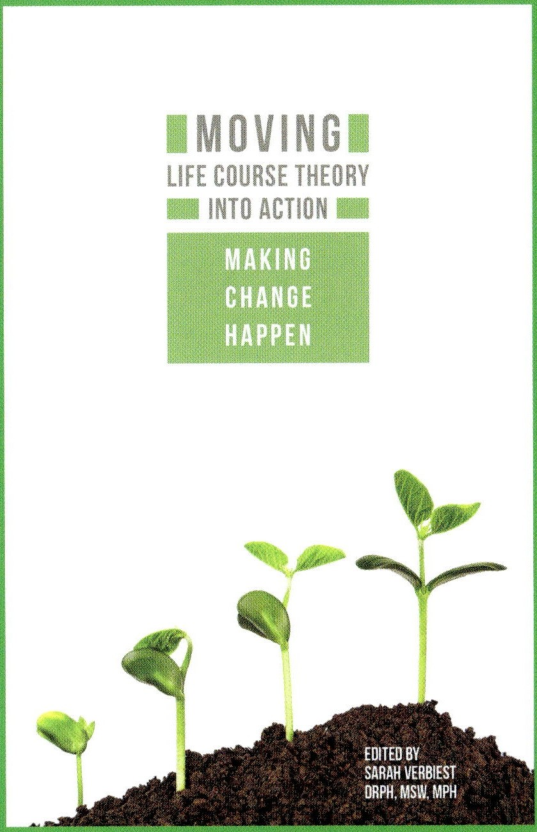

Moving Life Course Theory Into Action: *Making Change Happen*

Edited by Sarah Verbiest
DrPH, MSW, MPH

ISBN: 978-087553-2950
496 pages, Softbound, 2018

Over the past decade, practitioners in the field of maternal and child health have gained a general understanding of Life Course Theory and its potential application to practice. This book focuses on moving Life Course Theory into practice, thereby filling a need for practitioners across a variety of fields and providing them with valuable strategies on how to apply this approach.

Moving Life Course Theory Into Action is designed to fit into the busy lives of practitioners. With new ideas and strategies delivered in a compact handbook style format, each chapter includes key points that offer a quick summary of the main lessons advanced by the authors.

Order today at
aphabookstore.org

For classroom use contact
bookstoreservices@apha.org

APHA PRESS
AN IMPRINT OF **AMERICAN PUBLIC HEALTH ASSOCIATION**

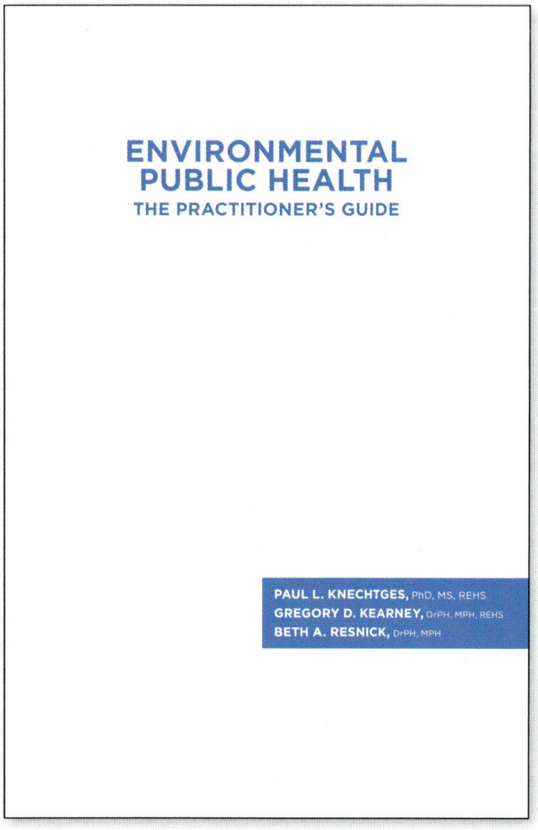

Environmental Public Health: The Practitioner's Guide

Edited by Paul L. Knechtges, PhD, MS, REHS
Gregory D. Kearney, DrPH, MPH, REHS
Beth A. Resnick, DrPH, MPH

ISBN: 978-0-87553-293-6
922 pages, softbound, 2018

The environment has a profound effect on public health and this new text not only covers the theory and science behind environmental health but also addresses real world issues faced by practitioners. The book's three parts present a clear picture of the problems with solutions for practitioners: the structure, major tools of, and finally programs and services for environmental health. The systems approach this work takes will equip the next generation of environmental health leaders with the tools to tackle the most challenging issues of our generation.

To purchase, visit **aphabookstore.org** or email **apha@pbd.com**

For review and exam copies, email **david.hartogs@apha.org**

APHA PRESS
AN IMPRINT OF **AMERICAN PUBLIC HEALTH ASSOCIATION**